Autobiographies of Our Orgasms

A Collection of Your Stories

Volume THREE

Edited by Betsy Blankenbaker

CONTENTS

DEDICATION

For each person who wrote to me after reading
Autobiography of an Orgasm but is still too afraid to
speak up – these stories are for you.

FOREWORD

From the moment I read Betsy's first book, **Autobiography of an Orgasm**, I was impressed with how important and essential her words were for me, my patients, and for women everywhere. Revealing the truths of our bodies creates a necessary path to breaking the cycle of silence and awakening the life force and powerful healer that resides in each of us - our orgasm. Her books, real stories from real women, show us the way. I knew upon meeting her that she and I were on a similar mission to help make the womb a healthier place.

Dr. Liz Orchard

Naturopathic Medical Doctor

Founder of Be Well Natural Medicine Clinic

www.bewellnaturalmedicine.com

NOTE TO READERS

This work is memoir. It reflects the author's present recollection of their lives. Certain names, locations, and identifying characteristics may have been changed. Dialogue and events have been recreated from memory to convey the substance and essence of what happened, but only represent the author's recollection of the events.

Chapter 1
SAYING YES
By Betsy Blankenbaker

I was born in Indianapolis, Indiana, also known as the heartland of the United States. If you think of the U.S. as a body, Indiana is roughly where the heart might be located. During the summers when I was a child, nearly every Sunday after church, we would drive 25 minutes to my see my maternal grandparents who lived on a 200-acre farm. I remember knowing how much was left of my summer vacation based on how tall the corn had grown.

My family had conservative, Christian values. My parents went to church, so I went to church. My parents believed in God, so I believed in God. My parents never talked about sex, so I never talked about sex. On the one occasion I can remember Mom talking to me about my genitals, she simply pointed and softly whispered, "down there" so you can imagine my mother's response when I released a book in 2014 called *Autobiography of an Orgasm*. She was not thrilled.

My book was about the five years I spent researching orgasm as a way to heal my body after sexual assault. When the book came out, Mom chose not to read it, and I understood why. "We don't talk about those things," she said. I could hear her mother and her grandmother and generations of women in my family - and in your families - saying the same thing: "We don't talk about those things."

Mom was a state senator in Indiana. She retired in 1992 after serving twelve years. She knows the risks of speaking up. In1992, her child support bill established requirements for the so-called deadbeat dads to pay child support, or their wages would be garnished. That night, a bullet shattered my mom's bedroom window—it landed just above where she was sleeping. But Mom continued to take a stand for the marginalized voices, especially women, children, and the elderly.

Mom modeled for me how to be positive and to think positive. The first time I saw her cry was when my dad died. I was twenty-five and she was fifty-five. If Mom ever cried before then, she didn't do it in front of me.

By the time I was thirty-five, I had a life that looked good. I was married with four children I adored. I smiled often, even though on the inside I was drowning in tears from not speaking up after sexual abuse and harassment as a child and teenager. I didn't realize that those unreleased tears were suffocating me until the rage I should have expressed years earlier became depression, and the judgment about my body and what I'd experienced often left me sick from all the toxic energy I kept inside. On the outside, I stayed positive. I said, "yes, yes, yes" during sex, even though I wasn't feeling a thing. When it came to orgasm, for more than half my life, I was smiling and faking it.

By the time I was forty, I could tell you all the words to my ten favorite songs. I could tell you in detail how to make my favorite dinner; I could tell you how to jump a dead battery on your car, but I couldn't tell you how to give me an orgasm. Finally, at the age of forty-five, I took myself on as a research project to see if I could feel my orgasm after a lifetime of feeling nothing.

First, I simply Googled videos on *How to have an Orgasm*. I do not advise that you do that—nothing that came up was helpful.

The next thing I did was read books called: *Easy Orgasm, The Elusive Orgasm, Extended Orgasm, Extended Massive Orgasm, Instant Orgasm, Real Orgasm, Tantric Orgasm* and *Super Orgasm*. The books were by lots of experts giving lots of advice. My head became full of too much information while my body remained silent.

I started to look for courses. I was living in Indiana and didn't bother to look for courses there—I would be too embarrassed to show up in a group and say, "Hi, I'm Betsy, and I'm trying to find my orgasm."

I wanted to do this research anonymously, so when I dropped my son Sam off at his first week of college in New York City, I signed up for a course on orgasm. No one would know me in New York.

I'd been a swimmer when I was younger, so I understood that I could train my body. I decided to quietly take up orgasm as my sport. I just had no idea if I'd be any good.

I signed up for a course to find my orgasm only to discover there was more than one kind. One course guaranteed the secrets to four types of orgasm. Another said nine. Another expert told me there were seventy types of orgasm. I was just looking for one.

I appreciated the wisdom of the experts, but the change for me came when I started listening less to the teachers and more to my body. Instead of the positive thinking I grew up with, I was listening for the positive feeling in my body, and I found my body was asking me to:

Go slower,

Breathe deeper,

Use my voice,

And know thyself.

As my research continued, it became less about orgasm and more about finding ways to keep my body in a balanced state of wellness—and that had nothing to do with sex. I found that I was really tracking the sensation that felt good, that was positive in my body, and then following the next positive sensation and then the next one. I was retraining my body to feel good. And then I started to do that in life, as well. I stopped doing the things in my daily life that didn't feel good or that felt like distractions. I stopped hanging out with people whom I thought were friends but really weren't. I found that saying no to things I didn't want was as important as speaking up for things I did want in my life.

The biggest surprise after five years of research? I'm the healthiest I've ever been. I am never sick. I'm the most creative I've ever been. And I'm the happiest I've ever been. Now when I smile, even my kidneys, lungs, and heart are smiling. I healed my body, not just through the medicine of orgasm but also by creating an orgasmic life and that has absolutely nothing to do with sex.

Recently, my mom called to tell me her book club started to read my book. "If someone wants to be in the club, they have to be open-minded," she said. She's eighty-four and I'm fifty-four. I guess it's never too late to have our sex talk.

Maybe it's time we talk about these things.

About the Author

Betsy Blankenbaker

www.betsyblankenbaker.com

Betsy Blankenbaker writes about sensuality, spirituality and self-realization. After releasing her first book, *Autobiography of an Orgasm*, something unexpected happened. Blankenbaker began to receive story after story from readers who thanked her for putting words to their own disconnection from their sensual energy. Her next books, *Autobiographies of Our Orgasms*, *Vol. I & II* became anthologies of reader's stories of the truth of their own sensual paths. The stories go beyond the physical to the emotional and spiritual experiences of being a woman. The storytellers, from Australia, U.K. and U.S., write with raw truth and transparency of the moment they listened to their bodies instead of the messages coming from media, church, family and partners about how sex should look or feel.

In her next book, *Beyond O,* Betsy discusses the consequences of speaking up in a culture where women's voices are frequently dismissed or cut off. Can telling our stories heal the lineage of women in our families who stayed quiet? Does liberating our voices lead to the liberation of our sensual energy and ultimate wellness and vitality?

Betsy teaches Qoya (www.qoya.love) and writing classes and retreats around the world. You can find out where she is teaching, or invite her to teach at your studio or event at **www.betsyblankenbaker.com.**

Chapter 2
GRIEF MEDICINE
By Kaci Florez

Two months after he left, I had yet to touch myself. I dreaded the emotion, the images, and the grief that orgasm would bring forth. Touching myself wasn't the problem. While he was here, I had become accustomed to self-pleasure. When your husband travels for two months at a time, it's essential. I happen to believe self-pleasure is essential even when you spend every night in bed with your partner, but it's even more important in the case of a traveling lover.

The first time I realized the importance of this practice was when we had been married only a month. Two weeks after our wedding, he had to go to Colombia, his home country, for a work project. He was going to break the world record for the longest wingsuit flight, and he had the help of the Colombian military to achieve this goal. At that point, there were few sponsorships, few jobs, and few paychecks. He was just a man with a dream and a deep love of flight. There was nothing I could do to stop him, nor anything I would do to get in the way of his passion. Between planning, press, and Colombian bureaucracy, his trip was about a month long. We were newlyweds and couldn't afford for me to take a month away from work, so I stayed home as he embarked on his goal. We spoke on Skype as often as we could, and while this helped ease the longing, it wasn't enough. My body craved his touch. I remember coming home after teaching yoga one day, and the craving was overwhelming. I had never felt anything like it before.

A couple weeks before our wedding I had been given a small, pink vibrator. It was a gift at my bachelorette party from a friend who knew what it felt like to have a traveling spouse. I remember laughing when I opened it, not really planning on giving it any use, but in this moment of deep yearning I recalled this pink gift. I found it in my underwear drawer, opened the package, inserted a battery, lay down on my back, and turned it on. I could feel the buzz of the pink tip before it even touched me. Then, at first touch, the pleasure was immediate and intense. I felt the orgasmic wave flood my body instantly, but I managed to prolong it before reaching climax. I inserted the tip a few times and envisioned my husband entering me. "My husband . . ." I hadn't gotten used to calling him that yet, and I already missed him. I fantasized about all the lovemaking we would do when he returned and all the places this would happen. I was grateful to know that even when he was gone I could connect with him through my self-pleasure and fantasies. I was grateful that these things were quenching enough until I could taste his skin again.

The trip and his time away was successful. He ended up setting four Guinness World Records. In a single jump, he achieved the greatest horizontal distance flown in a wingsuit, the greatest absolute distance flown in a wingsuit, the highest ever wingsuit jump, and the longest duration wingsuit jump—over nine minutes. These records kick-started his career in a way that nothing else had. His passion for flight was now his career; it forged our path as a young couple preparing to start a family. He traveled often, and sometimes I got to go with him, but even when I couldn't, we had Skype, and I had my fantasies to get us to our next time together.

About three years after my first experience with the pink vibrator, he had another trip. He would be training in Switzerland, competing in Norway, then back to Switzerland for more training for his next competition in China. When I dropped him off at the airport for that trip, it had begun to feel routine. We would wake up early, load his gear and the dogs in the car. I would drive. He sat with both dogs on his lap so he could soak up fifteen more minutes of puppy love. Then I would park at the curb, open the trunk, and he would unload his bags. I would get out of the car to give him one more hug and kiss before watching him roll his bags through the sliding glass doors. Then I would drive away, always conscious that every kiss could be the last. I would have a few tears and remember I had done this many times before. A few weeks from now, we would be returning to meet him at the baggage claim. The first thing he would eat would be a Chipotle burrito. Then we would go to bed that night with all our limbs entangled and my head on his chest. It was a beautiful routine and it was our life.

Over the years, my self-pleasure and fantasy life while he was away had evolved. I was no longer relying on the pink vibrator but took a softer and gentler approach with just my fingers. This allowed the process to last longer and be more intense. I had learned this technique from reading Betsy Blankenbaker's *Autobiography of an Orgasm* just a couple of months earlier, and my husband and I had practiced it together. He was fascinated and giddy when he saw how little it really took to give me pleasure. Not the pump and grind that movies and television portray. We had developed a sweet ritual together so that when he was away, to feel connected to him, I decided to use the same technique. I lay on top of my blankets and removed all my clothes. I wanted it to feel as unencumbered as possible. I also wanted to re-create as much of the setting as I could of him and me together. Every now and I then I would peek at myself in the vanity mirror near our bed, and I could see myself through his eyes. As I climaxed I felt him and eagerly anticipated when he would be home again.

We didn't get to speak as much on that trip. I was becoming busier with my own work, and his phone died on his way to Europe, so we were not able to talk as often or send messages throughout the day. I remember this bothering me, but instead of stressing about it I just counted the days for him to return. His travel had become common, and it had toughened me up a bit, so this lack of communication didn't get to me as much as it would have in trips past. He was set to return on July 8th, and it was already the 3rd. I already had my whole day planned out for the 8th. In fact, I had every day up to then planned. This schedule helped keep me occupied as I waited impatiently for him to return. I woke up on the 3rd to a Facebook message from him that simply said, "Hi baby." I wrote him back, knowing he was probably out jumping with no service.

I worked from the computer for a couple hours before going to a yoga class. He had purchased a local Swiss phone, so I tried calling a few times and received a recording in German. I didn't know what it said but figured he had run out of credit. I left him another message online and said I would be out of yoga in a bit and I couldn't wait to talk to him. When I got out of yoga there was no response. I went home and did a little more work from home. We were headed into the 4th of July weekend, which I would be spending with my family. I figured I would get a bit more work done, I would pack for the weekend, and then I would drive to my parents' house about twenty-five miles away.

For some reason, I felt a rush, like I needed to get to my parents' house in the early afternoon. But I was tired, so instead of pushing through, I decided to just take a nap. I still hadn't heard from my husband. Before lying down, I tried calling again, but no answer. This was a little unusual, but not totally unheard of as he was in the mountains, and often there is no reception. As I lay down with our two dogs, I laid my hands on my heart to ask God if he was okay. I remember feeling the answer as a long, soft "yessssss." But for some reason, I decided to ask again. This time I received no answer. Feeling a bit uneasy, I thought to myself, "Well, there is nothing you can do about it right now." I remember feeling like the nap would not only give me some energy, but it would help pass the time as I waited for his call. Then I fell asleep.

I awoke to my phone ringing. As I grabbed it off my nightstand, it said "unknown," which was common for international calls. For some reason, I knew it wasn't him. I picked up. "Hello?"

"Hi, Kaci, this is Felipe," my brother-in-law. He never calls me.

My heart started thumping, my mouth went dry, and I felt fire in my throat.

"Hold on a second," he said, "I'm going to get Camila on the phone."

Camila, their sister, got on the phone and says, "Hi, Kaci?"

"What happened?" I said in a deep, serious voice, bypassing any pleasantries.

She spoke slowly and had a hard time finding her words. I was getting impatient. I wanted to hear that she was calling about something minor, something unimportant. I was getting annoyed that she wasn't speaking fast enough to help get me out of this moment of worry and the uncertainty.

Finally she said, "Jhonny had an accident."

Confusion.

Why was she telling me this from Colombia when he was in Switzerland? If he had an accident, why didn't his jumping friends call me as he'd said they would if anything ever happened? I didn't believe Camila. I didn't want to believe her. I got mad.

"Where is he? What happened?" I wanted her to tell me what hospital he was at, what town he was in, and who was with him. I also wanted this to be a joke. A sick joke. I was getting mad at her for pulling such a sadistic joke. I couldn't wait for her to tell me she was kidding, and I could tell her how fucked up she was.

I don't remember much else of what she said but "He's gone."

Pacing, I began to ask questions for more information. She didn't have more information.

I had been awaiting his call that day. I realized that call would never come.

I remember screaming and crawling on the floor. I remember hitting the couch cushions. I remember what it felt like to be unable to comprehend the fullness of a piece of information I had been given. My husband was gone. That thought was too big to take in all at one time.

His call would never come.

I would not get to talk to him again.

I would not get to hear from him what was going on. I had so many questions that only he could answer. Only he could tell me the whole story. And I would never get to hear the story from him.

In the blur of shock and confusion during those first few moments of receiving the news, my next thought was "I never get to have sex with him again." The deepest and most intimate physical act. I'm not even sure if I had hung up with his sister yet when I looked at our bed and realized that we would never express our love through our physical bodies or give one another pleasure again.

I remember being a little surprised that this thought came to me so early on. Was I being shallow? Did it reveal a lack of depth to our relationship that I was lamenting our physical intimacy so early on? When I heard other people talk about losing their spouses I don't remember hearing sex being missed so quickly. Were they just holding something back? Was I just not hearing them? Was society not ready to hear them? Was this inappropriate to talk about? This was a moment that I felt the invisible expectations of societal norms and realized I could no longer pretend to fit within them.

He and I loved our physical intimacy, but our emotional connection was always the strongest part of our relationship. There were some days when we were both too tired to engage fully in sex. Rather than giving it a meager effort we would lie down, stare into each other's eyes saying how much we loved one another, and speak our hearts instead.

Two weeks after he passed I met up with another widow. Her husband, a friend of Jhonny's, had been gone for six years. I remember her saying that at three months the dildos started to show up. She said that's when she became so horny it was unbelievable.

It was two months out when I felt the urge to self-pleasure. I remember thinking, *this is too soon.* Something in me still thought there should be a timeline, a structure. I guess when our world crumbles, a part of us does wish for stable ground, even if the stable ground was simply knowing exactly when I would be horny again.

I remember having an insatiable need to climax. It was the middle of the day when I went to my room, closed the door, and got under the covers. I removed all my clothes. Already this was different than before. Prior to his passing there was no need cover up. But even in this insatiable state there were certain requirements I wouldn't compromise:

1. It had to be light. He and I favored making love at night under candlelight. When I touched myself, it couldn't be like that, so I did it during the day.

2. I needed to be under the covers.

I used to lie on top of the comforter when he traveled and I would imagine him with me or watching me anytime I would glance at myself in the mirror. This second requirement ensured that I wouldn't accidentally see myself in the mirror.

I lay under the covers and leaned over to open the drawer of my nightstand. Inside was the small pink vibrator I had been given at my bachelorette party. I turned it on and barely touched myself. Instantly I felt everything in my body turn on. I took my time penetrating a few times before touching my clitoris. It was so confusing. I had never felt anything that felt that good and that painful before. All my past experiences with this vibrator included fantasies about Jhonny entering me, kissing me, loving me. I would dream of the day of his return when we could make love again. This time my mind imagined him, but there was grief. He wouldn't be returning home to me this time. Before my fantasies were all fueled by anticipation. This time they were backed up by loss, grief, sadness, and confusion.

But here I was. As my heart ached, my body had decided what it needed, and it needed to climax. It needed *this* to feel this much. It needed this release, this rush, this oxytocin. I took my thoughts off Jhonny and my loss and just focused on the pure pleasure of sensation. With each breath, each touch, and each penetration, my genitals opened, softened, and celebrated. And climax I did.

In the post-orgasmic haze I remember feeling less sad than I had thought I would. I had imagined that orgasm would bring me into such pain that I would cry through the whole thing, then roll up in a ball of sorrow. But instead, it was healing. This physical act had been so closely linked to his body, and yet without his body present it still felt good. In fact, I felt better afterwards. It was an energetic release that helped me to move through my grief rather than get stuck. I did feel sadness that he would never give this to me again. But just like every breath connects us to our first and last breath, what if every orgasm connects us to our first and last? While I felt my loss, I also felt love and gratitude. It helped me to process some of the fears that I could not put into words.

Since then I have continued my journey with self-pleasure as a way to heal my grief, and I have found that my orgasm is a sacred medicine, holding divine wisdom and grace. I am not sure when I will be ready to receive this gift from another man, and this is why I am so grateful that I have chosen to give it to myself, and to receive all that this medicine has to offer.

About the Author
Kaci Florez

www.kaciflorez.com

What did you want to be when you were eight years old?

A country music singer

If you could give one piece of advice to your younger self about your orgasm, what would it be?

It's nothing to be ashamed of. There is nothing to feel bad about when exploring orgasm and your own body's sensations.

If your orgasm had a voice, what would your orgasm say to you about the piece you wrote for this book?

I am so glad you trusted me and let me help you.

Anything else you would like to add about your story or the experience of writing it?

This was a challenging piece to write as it required me to go back to the time and space that I was writing about. But it was also healing and empowering. I'm grateful because it gave me the courage and clarity to embark on writing my book.

Chapter 3
NO TRESPASSING
By Christine MacDonald

I've never been a rules person. Breaking any and all guidelines for being a good kid was my thing. Screw conformity. I'd scale the fence at the exact moment my brain registered the "No Trespassing" sign. If you told me I wasn't allowed to go there, I'd shoot you an adorable smile, nod obediently, and then do everything in my power to defy you.

Things began innocently enough. As a mischievous pre-teen, my adventures in search of complacency weren't very earth shattering. Days were spent dreaming of first kisses with Chachi Arcola from *Happy Days* and thoughts of navigating Rydell High School as both Sandy and Rizzo from my favorite movie, *Grease*. *There were worse things I could do.*

Every now and then my exploratory mind served me well. My impressionable brain was a delicious symphony of borderline dangerous adventure and idle curiosity. I possessed the perfect mindset to allow myself permission to experience things I never thought possible despite a brief church upbringing designed by our mother to keep my older sister and me in line. I don't know where the idea of religion started with Mom. Maybe not having a father in the mix for her two girls swayed her thinking. Instead of one dad to help her raise us girls she'd get the Father, Son, and Holy Ghost. Not that we were strict Catholics; our occasional Sunday Mass attendance was peppered with the usual holiday events each year. But that was enough. An hour of Mass, complete with accepting *the body of Christ* on my tongue while being reminded that He watches my every move was all I need to be freaked out. The long drives home served up haunting views from the back seat of Mom's station wagon. Hypnotized by the shimmering stained-glass windows framing the entrance to the church, I always wrestled with the pockets inside my breath.

Church visits stopped shortly after my thirteenth birthday when, after my first and only Confession, I decided the feeling of being wrong all the time just wasn't for me. Then there was the *why*. Why I felt the need to confess. And why I felt so guilty. Even though I was unconscious when it happened, I still thought I needed forgiveness for losing my virginity that night on the beach. I don't know what I expected to feel after releasing my truth bomb in the confessional, but it didn't make me feel any better. If anything, the blanket of shame wrapped around my shoulders became heavier. After the priest shelled out my Hail Mary and Rosary penance to absolve me of my sin (and what a doozy, at just 13), I walked away and never looked back.

Ever since I learned the difference between pink and blue booties I've been curious about my body. As a freshman in high school and shortly after the beach incident, my curiosities about sex grew stronger. One night when I couldn't sleep, I snuck downstairs to watch an R-rated movie on cable. After getting lost in this new wonderland of nudity and pleasure, my hunger for knowing the whys exploded. The next morning with the sun winking through the glass louvers in the bathroom, I sat on the toilet and opened my legs. Like a doctor asking me to say "Ah," I began to explore my vagina with my fingers. But it wasn't enough. I wanted to see myself, to visit the birthplace of the moans and pleasure scenes that had captured my attention the night before. So I ran to my bedroom, got my purse and scurried back to the toilet. I reached for the sliding door, ensured that it was locked, and grabbed my compact mirror.

Holy shit. I was in awe of *that place*—that sacred part of womanhood I was taught to never discuss. I loved every inch and fold of her. She was soft, fragile, and safely tucked away. But also, I knew she was a force. At some point, I moved from sitting on the toilet to lying naked on the floor. I opened my thighs and held the mirror with one hand, exploring myself freely with the other. My thoughts streamed together on a repeated loop of *wow, this is you* and *a baby comes through here—you can create life!* My very own **No Trespassing** sign.

The more I got to know myself, the more pissed off I became about that night on the beach at camp. Suddenly I didn't feel like my virginity was lost at all, but that it was taken. At just 13 years old, my No Trespassing sign was broken through without my permission. I wasn't even conscious!

That's it, I thought. *Never again.* It makes perfect sense that I faked my orgasms during my twenties. With each lover, I was an actress, making them think they rocked my world. Even if it weren't true, it was *my* lie and my body.

Behind closed doors and alone with my senses was another story. I enjoyed free-falling into pleasures beyond my control. Each orgasm was a love letter, a warm hug and high-five to myself. This is what it was all about—what sex should feel like. Not waking up in a tent with my bathing suit bottom rolled in a ball on the ground, covered in dried blood.

Never again. It was years before I would confess my secret to anyone but the priest. When I finally shared with Mom about the week I spent at camp and how her baby girl returned home a woman, the blanket of shame felt even heavier. I felt like that little girl being scolded in the confessional all over again, reaching for a life raft in her lungs, waiting for the stained-glass windows to fade.

It took a long journey of self-discovery to understand I was raped. Feelings of somehow bringing it on myself— *asking for it*— suffocated my self-worth, serving as landmines along the way. But I worked through that wreckage and got out from under the cloak of self-blame. And after much work on my own *whys*, the blanket of personal shame that suffocated my sanity for so long eventually disappeared. It has been replaced with something much lighter—an extension of me. The fabric is a delicate blend of strength and self-love. I've earned this survival cape and wear it with great pride.

Now in my forties, my presence with men is no longer forced and false. Trust no longer plays hide-and-seek with my fear. It is released within the space of freedom—freedom to let go and to know my body by allowing someone else to explore who I am. My No Trespassing sign is still intact, but I'm much more comfortable now, sharing the key that unlocks her.

About the Author

Christine MacDonald

www.poletosoul.com

"From working the pole to baring her soul."

What did you want to be when you were eight years old?

Ice skater (Dorothy Hamill) and superhero (Wonder Woman). Who wouldn't want to fly on ice while wearing magic jewelry?

If you could give one piece of advice to your younger self about your orgasm, what would it be?

Trust yourself enough to let go—with someone worthy of holding onto.

If your orgasm had a voice, what would your orgasm say to you about the piece you wrote for this book?

"Thank you for sharing our story. I knew we had it in us."

Anything else you would like to add about your story or the experience of writing it?

Working on this chapter for Betsy opened a new road for me personally and professionally. Working on my own autobiography, I've wrestled with thoughts on how to share my story about being raped at age 13. Aside from emotional road blocks, I tasked myself with orchestrating my voice in a very specific way. How do I write about childhood trauma without sounding weak? On the flip side, if I faced this piece stripped of vulnerability, I would seem callous and insincere. I wanted to pay tribute to Betsy, her vision and myself without sensationalizing or marginalizing the subject matter.

The heart of Betsy Blankenbaker's autobiography and subsequent anthologies are Orgasm. My autobiography is based on my lack of self-worth and the extraordinary choices I've made through the years as a result. It never occurred to me that both could be intertwined. After completing my chapter for Autobiography of Our Orgasms 3 (and with Betsy's invaluable guidance), this is the realization I never saw coming (no pun intended). Life is nothing without delicious lessons—and when they reveal themselves through growing pains born from passion, they taste even sweeter. I'm not only honored to share Betsy's pages with such phenomenal women, I'm excited to see where this new road of discoveries leads me with my own.

Chapter 4

REDEEMED

By Erica Wheadon

"You are not a healer," he spat. "You break men. You can't resist your patterns. Don't you ever. fucking. call yourself a healer."

I doubled over in pain, gasping for air, redemption, anything to stop the unholy chorus in my head that was latching onto his words and amplifying them. They sank into my brain like squid ink into a sponge.

Blackness. Everywhere.

The band around my chest grew unforgivably tighter.

I did not know this man. Or the snarl in his voice, the way he taunted me on the other end of the line, where he was safe. Where he didn't have to see the woman he claimed to have loved for a thousand years fall to pieces in a carpark, her shattered thoughts scattering on the ground, swept up in the thick swirl of humid air. The next wave of the storm would hit any moment. Instinct told me to move inside. Hang up and get to shelter. Leave him to his own madness. Walk away.

Thick heavy drops fell from the heavens. The type that can cover your face upon impact if you are staring at the sky, praying for redemption to a God you had not spoken to since you were

21. I didn't care who heard me. His words had done their damage.

My God. What had I done?

The past eight months flashed violently before eyes that were forced wide open in horror.

THIS is your reality now. I wriggled helplessly against its hold as perspective held me down.

The skies opened up as the regret swallowed me whole.

From the moment that we met, there was instant soul recognition. It was my first rehearsal, and I had been introduced to the other singers as they entered through the side door, curious about the new addition to the group. I stood nervously near the director. She was chatting to what seemed to be the only man in the room, who was leaning casually against the wall. He extended his hand towards mine. "Hi, Erica, I'm Tom. I'm the token male." I laughed and shook his hand confidently, desperate to make a good impression. Time seemed to come to a standstill as we looked at each other quizzically.

"Have we met before?" I asked.

"Possibly. I've worked with quite a few groups on the coast."

"No, I'm new to the coast. Have you always lived here?"

"For a while. Perhaps it was a workshop?"

"That could be it."

Despite our best efforts, we put it down to one of life's mysteries.

Before I continue, I feel that it's worth mentioning that I have always been flirtatious and largely sapiosexual by nature. I am also happily married to a man who doesn't have a single jealous bone in his body, who doesn't seek to possess me, harness me, or demand my love and affection, but rather gives me all the space I need to be myself. While I am the kind of woman who loves people deeply, the concept of forced monogamy confounds me, and I have never been fond of following rules blindly just because society demands it. It doesn't make me unfulfilled, or undisciplined, a slut, a whore, an adulterer, or any of the slanderous words that have been spat in my direction over the past 20 or so years. I simply vibrate with the energy of others around me. It's a primal need for connection and desire for awakening on all levels—mental, spiritual, and physical, particularly with men.

Despite this, nothing about Tom attracted me at all. The moustache made him seem older than his 47 years and he would walk into rehearsal with bare feet and faded t-shirts. He was convivial, chatty, and well-loved. He would talk about his partner's cooking and tell dad jokes. Not exactly what I'd consider intellectual catnip. As the weeks went on, I had expressed an interest in his arranging skills, and we had bonded over our almost identical tastes in jazz and '80s pop music, but that was where it ended.

Shortly after, the director of our group arranged a meeting to discuss the possibility of a new side project. I was excited to be included after such a short amount of time, and began excitedly discussing repertoire and prospective singers. When I casually mentioned Tom's name, her eyes darkened. I knew instantly that I had stepped over some kind of invisible line and that there was history between them.

Inwardly I groaned. I loathed group politics.

Still, curiosity alone was enough to pull my focus, and as I started to look closer, I began to notice little changes in the way Tom talked to me over the coming weeks. The way he'd stare at my hips from across the rehearsal room and lick his lips, just subtle enough for me to notice. Little messages of encouragement—always late at night and laced with enough flirting to get my attention, yet still indistinguishable to the naked eye.

A new professional collaboration opportunity had come up, and the week of the Easter eclipse had thrown us together on an empty beach, coffee in hand as he downloaded his entire life story to my open eyes and breaking heart. Any cynicism that I developed was swiftly pushed aside as I swallowed every word. His suicide attempt and the way he had clawed back to life, his affair and failed marriages, and finally the current relationship that left him completely unfulfilled. He'd never told anyone these things, of course. There was just something about me that drew it out of him, he said. I sighed. It wasn't the first time I'd been on the receiving end of such confessions, and yet I still had no idea how could I push away such a brave display of vulnerability. I looked into his eyes, usually so full of spark and positivity, now harrowed and wounded with the dark recollections of his recent past. I felt myself being drawn in, transfixed. Minutes passed, but it might as well have been a lifetime.

Damn it—where did I know him from?

It's hard to walk away when you've stared into someone's soul. The Tom that had laid himself bare at my feet was not the same barefoot family man who made us all laugh every Monday night. That mask had well and truly come off, and now that I had 'seen' him, there was apparently no going back. Emails of erotic fiction arrived in my inbox, punctuated with sad stories of missed opportunities and women who never understood him. The moustache disappeared. Daggy shirts were replaced with tight black t-shirts that clung to the physique of a runner who was well-read, cooked, and spoke French. My head was spinning at the rate of this unmasking, and gradually I felt less and less like I could resist the pull. Something had sparked within me and ignited into a small flame. A flame that I naïvely believed I could control.

As apprehension gave way to familiarity, he would begin to touch me lightly on the shoulder during our meetings, and I would feel a crackle of electricity arc across my body. Sometimes it was audible, and we'd stare at each other, bewildered but curious.

Insomnia kicked in, and I started to have visions of Bedouin tents and a dark man brutally taking me from behind, his hands pulling at my hair and my clothes, around my throat, draining the life force from me. Even more confusing, I had appeared to consent to this treatment and had not just welcomed but encouraged it. It wasn't long before the impromptu email fiction made way for a swarm of articles about esoteric theories. Twin flame. Twin soul. Instant sexual attraction. Fated. The words swam in front of my eyes as I struggled to make sense of it all.

Sleep became impossible as I became caught up in this rapidly unfolding mystery and memories that I didn't even realise I possessed. I'd have flashes of us together in both realities—and then flash-forwards to the three of us together. I looked at Cameron sleeping beside me and laughed a little despite myself. As openminded and supportive as he was, I couldn't ever imagine him signing up for that.

It wasn't long before the shoulder touches and hugs were replaced by kissing, which descended into rapid and unexpected acts of intimacy that would happen swiftly and take me by surprise. The concept of consent becomes foggy when your mind is a whirlwind. I mean, I didn't say no. Which obviously meant that I wanted it. Didn't I? Confused and consumed by a torrent of both guilt and fire, I would submit to his hands and his mouth, and after, he would smile triumphantly and softly whisper into my ear, "I'm not here to replace him. I'm here to set you free."

A balancing act began, borne of my addiction to his practiced hands and unholy tongue. Soon he had put an end to my doubt, swiftly and singlehandedly changing my taste in men and leaving me wanting more. More emails arrived in my inbox. More articles. The concept of polyamory made its way into conversation. "It's a legitimate theory," he purred. "I could never separate you two—you are simply inspiring to me. This is not an either/or situation. It's just we can't deny this connection, and it deserves to be explored."

He sent messages to Cameron describing how I was beauty and life and passion personified. How loved we both were. How he promised never to hurt me or our marriage. This is enlightenment, he'd state. Look at how fucking enlightened we all are. Cam stood by curiously as I spun into dizzying heights, consumed with something that can only be termed as madness. I was on fire. Self-righteous. Loved by two men and transcendent as fuck.

However Tom's double life caved in on him every time he returned home to his partner Josephine, who had been watching the man with whom she thought she shared her life withdraw and become more and more distant. She didn't know what was going on, only that I was involved, and she resorted to using every trick in her book, desperately fumbling to regain what she once had. I almost couldn't bear to watch. Another woman was being hurt through this deception, and while there was never any love lost between us, I never signed up for that. After a few weeks of attempting to trick Josephine into leaving him, he relented, put her out of her misery, and asked her to move out.

He did it for himself, he claimed, although we both knew that was a lie. He had never been alone. The concept frightened him, and as he was faced with his impending freedom, I'd open my door and find him broken and weeping, begging me to be his shelter and his sanctuary. I had recently rediscovered my healing talents, and I would pour my energy into his shaking hands and anoint his throbbing temples. The energy from our connection crackled to life and kickstarted a feedback loop, and I gave him an instant migraine instead, the mirror effect of our connection repeating ad infinitum. He looked at me. This is what it is to experience a connection with a twin flame. Did I see that now? I couldn't deny that I had no other explanation for it. I'd done energy work before, but I had never experienced anything as intense as that.

He wondered what it would be like to be in complete communion with me. Theoretically, he said.

We broke all boundaries before I was truly ready. He had me pinned down, poised, and promising that the decision was mine. For the longest time I believed it was. His hands gripped my hair. I reached out to the woman in the tent in my mind. She looked back at me with a dull, haunted sadness in her eyes.

For weeks I wandered around, lost in a reverie, walking between two worlds. Caught between the darkness and the light. I didn't know what was real anymore, just that we had a higher calling. A purpose. We were fated. Souls ripped apart by the cosmic fabric of time.

I wondered if we would begin to fray.

And then the moment of truth happened. The big revelation. The secret he had kept from the world. The secret he had kept from even me, his confidante. Tom didn't just love women. He experienced persistent longings to feel like one, revealing the shame at the hands of his mother, and secret addictions that disgusted him but that he couldn't walk away from. Boxes of satin and silk and lace would turn up on his doorstep one week only to be burned the next. I was numb. It's not that I didn't support the lifestyle or feel the pain of his admission, but he'd waited until he had had penetrated me on every level before he told me. Nagging feelings began to tug at the edges while I put the pieces together. His scorn and disgust for women was a mirror. What little rational mind I had left was begging me to untangle myself and get out while I still could, but I felt powerless. He was a broken, crumpled-up mess, and I felt compelled to take him in my hands and soothe him and promise that I would never leave. It felt like a familiar story, but I couldn't quite articulate why.

Soon, the man I had admired for his virility, his red-hot masculinity, his evocative words, his dominance and power and sexual prowess was falling under the weight of the magical worlds he had woven and betrayed by his own sleight of hand. He picked the wrong woman to sway and control. Instead, he had unleashed a wildcat who under his tutelage was on fire with possibility and all the ways she could revolutionise music and passion and joy. A woman who had started to speak up and take only what she needed. A woman who had begun to enforce boundaries.

Utterly emasculated, shrunken and soft, he would begin to make excuses. It was the whiskey. Lack of sleep. Here, let me set you aflame and distract you in other ways. I didn't want to be distracted. I could distract myself. I was an expert at distracting myself. I wanted to be fucked until my mind was not of this world. And then I wanted to get on with my day.

The night the three of us ended up together will weigh heavily on me as long as I live. It cannot be unwritten or rewound. It was the night Cameron and I allowed him into our bed, our sanctum. We had written the rules like that, so my marriage would stay intact and separate from our relationship, but somehow Tom had punched his way through our defences one night, and there we were, fumbling and tearing, hungry-mouthed until nothing remained but the ecstasy of being enfolded in the wet hot skin of two men who adored me. I breathed and believed that this could be true and real and possible. Tom smiled like a wolf who had been welcomed with open arms into Grandma's house in the woods.

I remembered the flash forward that I'd experienced at the beginning of it all and briefly pondered self-fulfilling prophecies.

Within the month, he had moved closer to where we lived.

"I know our agreement," he began as I started for the door. "I just can't bear to see you return to him. I just wish that you would stay longer. Stay, and I will make you food and feed you French wine and play you jazz and be your lover and . . . I can just pretend for a while that you're just mine. It's not fair that he has you all to himself."

"He doesn't," I would protest. I'd been there three days. I wanted my shower, and I wanted my bed.

We worked out a schedule that resembled more of a custody agreement than a contract between three consenting adults and creatively dodged questions from everyone who knew us. I didn't tell Cameron about the deep waters I had been treading or their dark undercurrent, preferring to focus on the professional part of our relationship. "We're building something. An incredible creative project, and it's going to be phenomenal. But he's going through some stuff. I need to stay for a few days." He agreed. There was no force in the universe that could stop me once I'd made up my mind, and he knew it.

He smiled and kissed me. "Whatever you need to do."

In the meantime, I tried everything to heal Tom. He spat darkness at me. I consumed it and still came to his door, oils and wine and music, my body willing to take whatever he could throw at it, whatever he needed to feel alive. Sometimes it worked. Sometimes it . . . almost worked. Sometimes he would lie there, his heavy arm across my body, pulling me in closer. His snuggling repelled me, and I felt trapped. This was not the intimacy I had signed up for. I signed up for fire, for life, for music, for cosmic communion. I signed up for everything in the brochure—not domesticity. I already had that. I was happy with that. I longed for the comfort of Cameron's arms. Of everything I knew before this madness began. The simplicity of my life before Tom arrived on the scene. A sleep without nightmares of masked men, desert women, and the ancient contracts between them.

Emotionally drained, I would redirect his attention. "Let's talk about the music. Or talk about our project. Can we focus on that for a while?" I'd suggest brightly, pulling out my notes.

He flatly accused me of wanting to leave him, of using him to advance my career. He'd shut himself away from me for days, cruel silence enveloping our plans. I never knew where he was. Where we were.

We flew to Europe for a research tour—a story in itself—and spent two weeks scratching and fighting and clawing over the tiniest indiscretions. I learned that the only way he could remain sexually potent was to hurt me. I let him. Over and over again. I took a private sabbatical to Spain and recalibrated my thoughts. It was the first time I'd had to myself in months, and I watched a fiery Andalusian sky fade to black, I knew deep down what was coming. We met up again in France, and the feelings that had taken root during our time apart had begun to grow. I swung violently between holding onto what we had and preparing for the end. As it turns out, I didn't have very long to wait.

Within weeks of being back, I learned of the suicide letter he had written me while I was sleeping next to him on the plane. A temporary madness had taken hold of him, and he was spinning out of control. We unravelled, faster than light.

By this time though, there was no light left. He was a shadow.

He was my shadow.

And he took no prisoners.

After the storm and the call that shredded what little self-worth I had been rationing at the back of my heart, I rocked back and forth, staring off glassy-eyed into space and bursting into tears every second. Blaming it on jetlag, I was holding a tidal wave of emotion behind the walls of my heart, and I was steadily, stoically refusing to let go.

I couldn't breathe.

It was my fault.

I broke this man. I break every man. I am not a healer. I am a breaker of men.

At home, Cameron couldn't reach me. I was catatonic and utterly resistant to his nurturing. Pushing him away was easier. I brought this on myself. I deserved everything I got, and more. He called in a friend to intervene, and I barely acknowledged her as I lay there, immersing myself in the white noise of my own grief. She took my hands and looked me in the eyes and used words like abuse.

Fear. Obligation. Guilt.

He has been gaslighting you for eight months.

Listen to me.

Listen.

Trust my hands. Trust my heart. Trust the concern in my eyes.

I don't know what it was, but just as I was sinking under, something made me grab onto her rope and begin the steady climb back to life.

It took almost another eight months until I found the courage to face Tom again in a cafe close to his new house. After finally agreeing to meet, he looked into my eyes, and held my hands, fighting back tears, and he told me that he would never forgive himself for ruining my life. For hurting Cameron. For being selfish and knowingly trying to come between us.

My fear dissipated. He was just a man.

Instantly my heart softened. "Then I will forgive you instead."

I silenced the cries of horror from my friends. It was my decision. And I chose to take the high road. It was my sin to forgive.

It took two weeks for him to do it to me again.

This time, however I sought help from shamanic healers and Akashic record readers who helped me to understand the nature of soul contracts. I traced back through past lives and spoke softly to every version of myself that had felt powerless against his grip. I consciously distanced myself from the twin-flame theory that was binding my memory to his and cautioned others against using the same label. This was not the same thing as a soulmate. It was a disempowering, unproven, mythological excuse to put up with abusive, narcissistic behaviour, and I was done.

I committed to my recovery and loving myself like it was my job.

I wrote, voraciously, every day.

And then one morning—out of nowhere, purely without any kind of flourish or fanfare—I decided to forgive myself. I realised in this moment that this entire experience had made me stronger and more sure of my identity not only as a woman, but also as an artist, teacher, and healer. I still vibrated with the fire of connection with others—but I had learned to do so with stronger boundaries.

Prior to this revelation, I had allowed him to become the regret beneath my guilty skin, the knives I would turn upon myself on my darker days, and the voice of hatred and disgust in my head. He was dormant in the thick silence when Cameron and I spoke of the year we lost, in the way our voices would trail off, in the hand I would place on his cheek, the tears in my eyes, the unspoken words: I'm sorry. God I'm so sorry.

But he also became the fire in my belly, the prologue to narratives still unwritten.

Only I could write its ending.

And it is only through the power that I have bestowed upon myself that I am redeemed.

About the Author

Erica Wheadon

ericawheadon.com

What did you want to be when you were eight years old?

I was encouraged to either become a doctor or marry one, but secretly I wanted to be a performer.

If you could give one piece of advice to your younger self about your orgasm, what would it be?

Let no boy, no man, no soulmate, no sacred text nor passing belief dictate what you know deep down to be true.

Anything else you would like to add about your story or the experience of writing it?

I wanted to resist every word, every scrap of this story as it poured out of my hands. Wracked and consumed by guilt, I was terrified of the impending walk of shame that would inevitably follow its unleashing into the wild. It was then that I considered the two best pieces of advice about writing that I had ever been given. The first was by Ernest Hemingway, who implored all of us to write the truest sentence we know.

The second, from William Chapman who wrote: "If you can touch one heart with what's in yours, you were not only meant to be a writer, you are obligated."

The time for shame has passed. It is not a threat, and it can no longer be used to hold us for ransom while those who strip us bare rejoice in their arrogant victories. There is nothing more dangerous than a woman who is naked and unashamed, clawing at the bindings around her wrists, fire and rage in her eyes. These wolves who favour sheep's clothing claiming to be evolved, pro-feminists, who bleat convincingly about loving kindness and and yet continue to do untold damage in places where no-one will see and ensure that we will never be believed? Their time has passed. And with every word we find the courage to write, publish, rinse, repeat, we peel the mask back inch by inch and expose their narcissism to the light, a place impossible for it to hide, or survive.

Together, we are stronger. But together out loud, we are free.

Chapter 5

LATE BLOOMER

By Hannah Smith

I wish we encouraged young girls to pay attention to more than how their bodies look. What if a girl knew to listen to her body's internal messages, especially when she chooses to become sexually active?

I discovered my genitals by the time I was four years old, and I frequently enjoyed touching myself because it felt good. I felt a release from the tension and fear in my body, and I felt momentary pleasure. It took me somewhere else. It was a time I could feel anything other than the numbness. I felt numb because there was no physical affection or emotional connection in my childhood from my parents or any other family members. There was a lot of fighting and screaming, and the only way I could survive at that time was to go numb. I was told I often rocked as a baby in my crib, and it wasn't till I majored in psychology in college that I learned the rocking was my way of self-soothing, and I suppose the masturbation was a way, too.

When I became sexually active in my twenties, the same body that had felt so good in my own hands experienced dryness and tightness with my partner. Even when it was painful as he tried to penetrate me, I didn't stop him. Instead of taking it as a message that maybe he wasn't right for me or that I needed to guide him in his lovemaking, I decided that something was wrong with me.

Shortly after we began having sex, I visited Planned Parenthood to get birth control for the first time and was given a pelvic examination. I will never forget the look on the nurse's face as she completed the exam and looked at me with such sadness. She said, "You have genital warts."

It was 1994. It wasn't referred to as HPV then, a term that has a much less horrific visual attached to it than genital warts. After I found out about the HPV, I felt my sex life was over because who would want to touch me now? I was stuck in a mindset of feeling damaged as there is no cure for HPV. I wondered if my partner had any other diseases, and my mind wandered to the fact that I had taken his word that he didn't have any sexually transmitted disease.

When I told him that I had HPV, I was away at college, and he was three hours away. I was devastated. He claimed he didn't know he had HPV at that time. That evening we talked on the phone, and he told me he had to go because he was attending a music concert. I remember crying uncontrollably, feeling like my sex life was over. I didn't reach out to anyone because of the shame.

I began having a host of symptoms and went through numerous tests. One day I was in my OB/GYN's office, and he said, "Many of your symptoms are indicative of HIV. Have you had a test?" I almost fainted.

I waited nervously several weeks for the answer. During that time I felt deep shame and wondered how I would survive a disease like this along with the stigma. I was too ashamed once again to reach out to any of my friends for support. My boyfriend kept reassuring me he had been tested, but that obviously gave little consolation.

I found out I didn't have HIV, I had another disease that has many of the same symptoms. I eventually began vomiting blood and was taken to the emergency room, where my white blood cell counts were so elevated that I had a bone marrow test the next morning. The day after that, a doctor came into my room at 5:00 a.m. I was alone, and he preceded to tell me I had leukemia in the most matter-of-fact way. At this point my body was beginning to shut down, and I barely understood him. I wasn't surprised, though, because I knew I was slipping away. It had been almost a year of not feeling well and countless tests before I was diagnosed with leukemia. On some level, I felt relief to know there was something really wrong. I had been told it was "all in my head," so it felt good to get validation of what I'd known all along—that something was seriously wrong with my body.

I stayed with the same man from whom I contracted the HPV during the year-long treatment for the leukemia. He continued to pressure me for sex, and I continued to oblige. I am 5'6" and weighed about 97 pounds during the treatment. I lost all my body hair and was on hormones to stop my periods, as I was at risk for bleeding out. The chemo I received was so strong there were barely enough platelets for my blood to clot. The doctors told me that the strength of the chemo meant my chances of having children would be very small. My body was barely existing. I had to stay in a hospital room for six weeks and was not allowed to leave that room the whole time; I was at high risk of hemorrhaging and contracting an infection that would be lethal because I had no immune system.

After the six weeks in the hospital, I was allowed to come home for four weeks, when my body was supposed to recover enough to go back in for more chemo. I did this cycle of six weeks in the hospital and four weeks at home three times. I remember at night I looked in the bathroom mirror and cried, asking God if he wanted me to live through this. I would do whatever it was He wanted me to do while here. I don't know why I stayed with my boyfriend at that time—I think he was one more thing I couldn't bear letting go of, and frankly, I don't think I was in my right mind. I was just trying to not die at the time.

One month after the treatment was completed, he went down on me, and I contracted herpes because of a cold sore in his mouth. My body couldn't scream any louder to stop being with this person. When I suspected I had herpes, I went to my OB/GYN, and she looked at me. I know she meant well, but she said, "When will you learn to stay the hell away from this man?" At the time, I was broken in so many ways, and her comment brought more shame. My boyfriend admitted at the time that he had given a previous girlfriend herpes, and it had ended their relationship. It still took me several months before I finally ended my relationship with this man. I couldn't stand it when he touched me; I couldn't stand the sound of his voice or even his smell, but I still couldn't let go. I didn't think I deserved better, and I was afraid he might be the only one who would be with me because I was stained now.

Sometimes after cancer people shed their fears and live fearlessly. I went the opposite direction. I had always been fearful, but then, after being diagnosed with HPV, then almost dying from leukemia, and then discovering I had herpes, I was just waiting for the next crisis to happen. I didn't trust my body—or anyone else, for that matter—and worst of all, I didn't trust my own intuition. Self-love was clearly absent.

Through my twenties and thirties, I just pushed my way through life. I had a few short-term relationships during those years. Without the self-love, it was always just sex. Truthfully, I wasn't often present—I just "checked out," which I was so good at doing in my life. I will never forget the time a man said to me after I told him about the STDs, "You know, they have a dating website for people with STDs. Maybe you should try that."

On the flip side, I had a few men say to me after I told them about the STDs, "Me too," and I could tell it was just as distressing for those particular men. While they didn't verbalize it, I could feel their shame. They feared being judged as unworthy of being touched—or maybe I was projecting my own feelings onto them.

Sex never included oral anymore, and I understand why, but that didn't mean my desire for it left. I long for a man to go down on me. To feel his tender lips on my pussy. To be so vulnerable as to have someone breathe me in and taste me. To me, this is so much more intimate and vulnerable than intercourse. I understand completely why a man wouldn't want to go down on me because of the risk of oral herpes or HPV. Truthfully, I haven't let go of the shame, because even if a man wanted to use a dental dam, I still feel like I have something dirty I could pass on.

I didn't even like to insert my own fingers into my pussy, because I felt like it was unsafe. There was no more masturbation, and my pussy and sensuality faded, along with creativity, joy, and on and on. I associated sexual intimacy with getting sick.

The thoughts that ran through my head . . . Could I give my partner an STD even though we were using protection? Could I be allergic to the condom? Could I get a UTI? Never mind if I even enjoyed it—I worried about whether it could make me ill. If he goes too fast or too hard, could my pussy or my insides get hurt? Will my cervix bleed? Why am I not using my voice and talking about all my fears beforehand—because it is a mood-killer? Why am I not with individuals who will engage in these discussions? Maybe I had been and just didn't initiate them.

About a year ago, I had sex, but again it was the disconnected kind. I left his home the next morning and walked into the shower. As I was washing myself and the water ran over me, cleansing me, I just knelt down and cried. I hugged my body. I kissed my body. I told my body how sorry I was for not protecting it, for not loving it, for not setting boundaries. All of a sudden, it all clicked how everything in my life was not okay because I wasn't saying NO. I wasn't speaking my truth, I wasn't setting boundaries for myself or my body. My body had been through so much, yet it was still always there for me, trying to communicate what it needed or didn't need.

My journey of releasing my fear, my victim mentality, and mostly importantly my lack of self-love has taken place during the last year. These life experiences and the story I have woven around them will probably continue changing, but the one core theme is self-love. If you read this and walk away wanting to look more closely at the depth of your self-love, then I will feel that I didn't share my story in vain.

Be love, but be love to you first.

Note from Editor: In the U.S., with STD diagnoses higher than ever, most STD cases continue to be ignored, which can lead to further health complications. Thank you to Hannah for bravely sharing her story, so others can be responsible for their own health and wellness.

About the Author

Hannah Smith

What did you want to be when you were eight years old?

I wanted to be a teacher. I always saw myself talking with people. I am not even sure about what, but I know I felt this sense that I was trying to protect others in some way.

If you could give one piece of advice to your younger self about your orgasm, what would it be?

It is yours, Dear One. It is all yours. It isn't something you give away or wait till someone else gives you. It is safe, and it is an expression of all that you are.

If your orgasm had a voice, what would your orgasm say to you about the piece you wrote for this book?

I never meant to hurt you. I only wanted to free you in so many ways. There is so much I still have to give to you, to open you up to. Don't give up on me as I will never give up on you.

Anything else you would like to add about your story or the experience of writing it?

Writing my story helped me to realize how much pain I am still carrying in my body. This I see as a positive awareness, and it will help me to release and move forward despite not knowing what that will look like or involve. Another positive: it wasn't till I wrote this piece that I became clearer on what I desire. I have accepted the fact that my soul—and especially my body—prefer soul intimacy prior to bodily intimacy. This may mean a long getting-to-know-you stage with sensual touching and kissing. This stage will likely be longer than what many are accustomed to, but this is needed for both my lover and myself to move forward consciously, lovingly, and tenderly towards sexual intimacy. Making love in this way can be just as erotic as the act itself. Before we make love, I want to look into a man's eyes and know what he is communicating. I want to know his scent, the way his breath changes when he is turned on, the way he licks his lips when he is wanting to kiss. All of these idiosyncrasies are part of making love. The key to this is that I have to be vulnerable with someone, and honestly, I don't know if I am there yet—the operative word being yet.

Chapter 6
THE MASTURBATION DIET
By Rebecca Clio Gould

In the winter of 2015, I was struck with a brilliant idea: to masturbate any time I had a craving for junk food, like ice cream or chocolate. That's right. I kid you not. My thinking was that it could help prevent me from emotional eating, especially if I was feeling lonely, anxious, or blue.

I mean, if my cravings were coming from a part of me that wanted to feel pleasure, connection, and fulfillment, why not reach down and touch myself rather than reaching for a pint of Ben & Jerry's or devouring an entire chocolate bar? I figured some good self-lovin' could be just as effective, if not more so, in making me feel satisfied.

But allow me to back up for a moment. This stroke of genius didn't exactly come out of nowhere. It came shortly after a trip to Bali that inspired an even bigger idea.

While traveling around, I'd been thinking a lot about what it means to live fully alive and how to fill up on the pleasure of life. And on the flight home, I suddenly started getting what felt like a creative download, and the words "write me now" whispered in my head. I obeyed and started filling the pages of my journal with an outline for a book about cultivating sexual energy, sensuality, pleasure, and self-love. And this book wanted to be called . . . *The Multi-Orgasmic Diet.*

I almost ended up calling it *The Masturbation Diet* instead. Why? Because of that idea I'd had about masturbating to help me out with my sweet tooth. It also occurred to me that by masturbating before each meal, or at least once a day, I just might make healthier food choices in general and experience a greater sense of overall well-being.

I started wondering if masturbation, with or without peak orgasm or climax, could be the answer for any and all problems in life. Why not? It feels good, it's a way to experience pleasure regardless of the other things happening around you, and it doesn't require a partner or money.

And so it began. I decided to commit to this new daily practice. For two weeks, I'd either start my day with getting myself off, or whenever a craving for something like ice cream arose, I'd take myself into the bedroom instead of out to the store.

Within the first couple of days, I noticed that I felt happier, more energized, and was radiating a healthy glow. But what about the impact on compulsive or emotional eating and cravings? Check this out . . .

For years, I had this habit of eating my parents' chocolate from Trader Joe's every time I visited them, even though I didn't really like it. Nevertheless, there was always this magnetic pull I experienced when going back to my childhood home—like functioning on autopilot as I walked into the kitchen and opened their chocolate-filled cabinet.

But thanks to my Masturbation Diet experiment, guess what happened that first week? I didn't feel the pull while visiting. I didn't even think about that chocolate. For the first time in years, it wasn't a struggle to avoid it. I simply made it through the visit without any urge or impulse for chocolate, because I felt such a deep sense of satisfaction and connection with myself and with the universal, sexual energy that was filling me up. I wasn't yearning for anything unhealthy, and so without even trying, I broke the habit just like that.

It was working! Until I got to a point of "not being in the mood." So I realized that masturbation and reaching climax could help, but it wouldn't really be sustainable as a daily practice. And that got me wondering about the essence of what was really going on. How could I make myself feel sexually vibrant and fulfilled even when not having sex, either with someone else or with myself?

I started taking some time to just love myself up more, whether through sweet caresses, eye-gazing in a mirror, or things like taking myself out on a date. Sometimes I still use masturbation when a craving comes on. But sometimes I just look in the mirror and smile at myself, and that helps me feel full of love, more content, and less likely to overindulge or give in to unhealthy cravings. Now I know that although there is plenty of healing and magic in orgasm, there are other ways to feel some of the pleasure and other benefits that orgasm brings. In fact, I even started to redefine orgasm as "the pleasure and pulse of life," thereby making more of my everyday life feel *orgasmic.*

Now, instead of being hungry for the pleasure of sweets, I nourish myself with the sweetness and pleasure of self-love and awakened senses. Rather than reaching for Ben & Jerry's, I reach down and touch myself or go outside to breathe in the delightfulness of the fresh air against my skin, the earthy and fragrant smells of nature, the beautiful sights all around me, and the sounds of the birds chirping. With each breath, I feel my heart expand and a wave of pleasure wash over me. I am full.

Editor's Note: A version of this story originally appeared in *Elephant Journal*.

Chapter 7
THE FANTASY TRAP
By Rebecca Clio Gould

The first orgasm I ever had—with someone other than myself—was with my now ex-husband. But I was fantasizing about someone else. It's not that I wasn't attracted to my ex. It's not that I didn't love him. But I had spent *years* having orgasms without him, and oftentimes while fantasizing about one of my high school crushes—let's call him Jake. Thoughts of Jake had become my orgasm crutch; I needed to think of him for that final orgasmic peak and for release to happen.

I met my ex (let's call him Brian) while still in college and still in contact with Jake. I hadn't had much sex, other than with myself, prior to meeting Brian. I was a virgin until I was twenty, and I'd never had sex with anyone with whom I was in a "real relationship." I just had a few flings, Jake being one of them. I hoped that with Brian, because we saw a future together, I'd be able to fully let go with him, *without* fantasizing. But I was wrong. Perhaps it shouldn't have come as a surprise, but it did.

I remember us going at it on a mattress on the floor of his living room. The lights were off, but the TV was on, and the video for the Enrique Iglesias song "Hero," was playing. The feeling of skin against skin and sweet kisses felt good as I rubbed my wet pussy against his hard cock. I knew how to get off, and at that time in my life, it needed to happen prior to penetration, by rubbing up against something to stimulate my clit. But I'd actually experienced it only a couple of times with other men. Mostly, I'd just been giving myself orgasms for years. I don't know if it was the music or the self-imposed pressure to reach climax combined with self-consciousness, but I just couldn't get there that night with Brian—until I shut my eyes and imagined I was with Jake. And then, suddenly, I was no longer wondering or worrying about was happening or not happening. I was gyrating and undulating on auto-pilot as ripples of pleasure flowed through me. I remember laughing at the ridiculousness of the soundtrack and the words when Enrique sings "I can be your hero, baby" and how perfect it was in a way, since fantasy Jake had just been my hero, saving Brian and me from mediocre sex.

I was young and sexually inexperienced at the time. I didn't read too much into it that first night, but I did feel a little bad about thinking of Jake in order to climax with Brian. I didn't try to change it or stop myself; Brian was so happy that I came, I didn't want to let him down. I didn't have the skills to be fully present and surrender into orgasm with Brian, so I continued to do what worked: think of Jake, even just for a few seconds in order to cum. Although Brian was the man who made my heart melt and who wanted to spend his life with me, thoughts of Jake were what got me off pretty much every time during the first year we were together. Maybe that's because it's hard to break a habit. In true Pavlov's dog fashion, my yoni, my clit, were hooked on Jake. After all, I did have a long history of fantasy with him.

I could tell you various stories about my interactions with Jake over the years, most of which felt like foreplay and had me addicted to what I couldn't have in reality. But this is one of my favorites: the power-struggle phone call shortly before the one night we finally had sex.

It was the summer of 2000, and I was home from college in my very own apartment in downtown Seattle. I was hoping Jake and I would finally have a chance for a little summer fling after years of sexual tension. But when I called him earlier in the week to invite him on a little road trip down to California, he said, "I'd love to, Rebecca, but I can't. I've gotta work like a dog every day of August."

I could picture him waking at five o'clock every morning, determined to spend all day either working as a carpenter or skateboarding. I let it go without a fight, but a few minutes later I recalled several times when he had tried to corrupt me, giving me a hard time about being too level-headed and moral for my age, and so I decided to give it back to him.

When I called back, I got voice mail and left the following message:

"Hi, Jake, it's Rebecca again." Pause. "Ya know, it occurred to me that if *you* were to invite *me* on a road trip, and I told you, 'Oh, I'd love to, but I have to work,' you'd give me that carpe diem crap, and tell me to 'go for it,' 'have fun,' 'fuck work.' And maybe you don't have that type of attitude anymore. Maybe you can't afford to be that carefree right now, but, uh, I dunno . . . Think it over."

It took him awhile to return my call, and I thought maybe I had frightened him off for good this time, but he did call, a couple days later. Not frightened off. Even reminding me of his number, telling me to call, as if I didn't have his number, as if I might not call.

I listened to his message in my car, in a parking lot, sleepy before returning home after an afternoon spent with an old friend. Hearing his voice made my heart stop, pause, and then speed up. Now I was awake. Now I was beaming, and with a lingering smirk and some recurrent giggles, I raced home to return his call. I don't remember much about the drive back to my place other than looking at the clock every couple of minutes, wondering if Jake would still be home or awake.

And when I walked into my apartment, the combination of heat, stuffy air, and vanilla-scented candles nearly knocked me unconscious. I started taking off my clothes as I headed straight for the porch door to let in some fresh air. I put on some shorts and a tank top and plugged in my little plastic fan. I went to the bathroom and pulled my hair up on top of my head, got a glass of water and applied some lip balm. Then I sat down on the edge of my couch with phone in hand. Took a deep breath.

Dialed his number.

He said, "Hello."

"Hi!" I leaned back, relieved to get hold of him.

"Hello? Hello?" he said, as if he couldn't hear me.

"Jake," I said, figuring he was messing with me. He chuckled, and I knew that he knew, but I played along and said my line anyway, "It's Rebecca."

"Rebecca!" he inhaled. "What's up, Gould?" And then he exhaled, "I got your message."

"Yeah." I smiled.

"Yeah," Jake continued, "Did I call you back?"

My face scrunched up, and I let out a gasp of confusion. "Whaddya mean? That's why I'm calling you. You don't remember calling me back earlier tonight?"

"Well, I got your message on Friday, and I couldn't remember if I had called you back when I got it—"

"Jake," I interrupted, in response to his nonsense. "Are you high?"

"No."

I laughed at him and told him that he hadn't called me until tonight. And then somehow we ended up taking a detour through the land of small talk. He told me all about his week, and I told him about my man troubles and the movie *But I'm a Cheerleader.* I don't remember which one of us got back on track, but it didn't take long before we were talking about my road trip invitation.

Again he told me, "I can't. I gotta work."

"And you can't take two or three days off?" I looked up, as if I were waiting for a message from the heavens above.

Instead, Jake said, "Two or three days would be a lot of grocery money down the drain."

"Party pooper."

"Gould."

I looked around the room searching for the right words, "Well what if you were sick and needed to take time off?"

"I work when I'm sick."

"What if you were bedridden or injured, and the doctor told you that you couldn't work for a few days?"

"Like if I had a hernia or something?" he sounded hopeful.

"Yeah, now you're getting it. Why don't you just look at it like that?"

"I don't know. I just don't know if it can happen."

"C'mon Jake," I encouraged, "make it happen! You can do it!"

"Rebecca?"

"Jake?"

"Why do you want me to go with you?"

Gulp. Moment of truth. I immediately got wet but then started babbling. "Well, I think it would be fun, really fun. I just think it would be fun. Don't you?" I silently laughed at myself for sounding like such an airhead on speed.

"I do. I think it would be fun, too," Jake cleared his throat, "but Gould, I want to know why you want this so badly. I want you to tell me why you, Rebecca Gould, want me, Jake Thompson, to accompany you on your venture. That's what I wanna know."

What he really wanted was for me to declare my undying lust for him.

My world froze into a sort of meditative state while I negotiated with myself about things like my pride. I hated it when he did this to me, but after considering our past, my present state of mind, and my imaginary future, I felt that I really had nothing to lose. Why not bare it all?

But I said nothing until provoked again.

"Rebecca?"

"Jake," I shifted my weight and drank some of my water, "why do I want you to go with me?" I paused, trying to muster up the courage to be honest, and then continued, "Well, I think you'd be incredibly entertaining, and we would both learn a lot and have a great time. And maybe we'd finally finish what we started during winter break, but even if we didn't, it would still be fun. I feel like no matter what might happen, or *not* happen, it would be okay. It wouldn't be weird or awkward, ya know?"

"Yeah, I totally feel that."

I nodded my head as I imagined he might be doing. "It may sound a bit odd, but I can just picture it. I can picture it happening, you and me on a road trip, driving around, figuring out where to stop along the way—"

Jake interrupted, "Finding some nature spot where I can dance around naked, and you can laugh at my white ass."

I was tickled by that image, and then he asked, "What else can you imagine? Tell me what you've been daydreaming about."

"A cheap motel room." Surprised by how fast and easily that came out of my mouth, I bit my lower lip and slid off the couch onto the floor.

Had I really said that out loud?

"Cheap motel!" Jake repeated. "Who needs a motel room?"

"Fine, Jake. Ruin *my* fantasy!" I tried to come up with one he might like better, and in an exaggerated, sultry voice, I asked, "How about a tent? Would that do it for you?"

"Maybe, Gould, but why don't you go ahead and tell me what happens in that motel room?"

I lay down with my feet up on the couch, and I entered into my rich inner world full of cheap motel rooms. This time the lighting was dim, and the room had that sort of '70s gold, brown, and orange decor.

Jake really knew how to bring out the best in me, didn't he?

"C'mon, Rebecca. What are you thinking?"

"No, Jake. I'm not gonna take you there right now."

"Why not?"

"I've told you before: I'd rather show than tell. You yourself have even advocated that show-don't-tell philosophy."

"But I was referring to your writing style. C'mon, Rebecca. Talk dirty to me."

My eyes widened, and I sat upright. Jake knew perfectly well that I would never go along with this, and my reply was a melodramatic, "No way, you creep!"

"Just repeat after me," he said, "'Oh Jake, I want your cock.'"

I burst out laughing. Did he really think I'd say that? I was practically still a virgin. But I wasn't. Just a late bloomer. And inhibited.

"Rebecca," he pleaded.

"Fine." I called forth my most sarcastic monotone voice and repeated, "Oh Jake, I want your cock. There, I said it. Happy?"

"Yeah."

"But I said it with absolutely no feeling. They were just words, and they weren't even my words. They were your words. Don't you think it would be better if they were my words?"

"All I think, Gould, is that you just need to explore this more."

"Well, I think you don't really need my help to get off right now."

"Are you telling me I should go masturbate?"

"If you're not already, Jake."

He laughed.

I rolled my eyes but smiled. "I'm not gonna do it. You'll just have to go on this road trip with me if you wanna hear me talk dirty and find out what I've been cooking up inside my lil' ol' head."

"I'll tell you what, Gould."

"What?"

"I'll call my boss tomorrow and see what I can do."

"Oh, goody," I teased. I was proud to see that my attempted persuasion was working.

"But tell me one more thing, Rebecca—"

I sighed. "What? What now?"

"What's the deal with this guy you've been dating? Why didn't you invite him?"

"I don't wanna talk about him. He's great. He's affectionate, intelligent, attractive, funny, reliable. He's everything that I thought I wanted, but I'm not turned on by him. I don't know if it's because he looks kind of like my brother or if being with him has made me think a lot about my past relationships. I don't know. The whole thing has sort of weirded me out because I've realized just how badly I've been treated in the past, even by you."

"What did I do?"

"Hmmm. What did you do? Well, there was winter break. You called me, at the very moment you should've been ringing my doorbell to take me to a movie, to tell me that you had changed your mind about your proposition for 'one night of passion.' And back in '95, when I was a bold freshman who invited you, a hot senior, to Spring Tolo, you stood me up."

"I stood you up?"

"Yeah! Duh?! Don't you remember? We've talked about this before. I even reminded you about it during winter break, and you said you'd take me out and make it up to me," I mimicked him and sat down on the couch again.

"Gosh, Gould, I don't remember. I've actually been thinking a lot about that time in my life and what a horrible person I was, but I don't remember standing you up. That's really bad."

"You were smoking too much pot back then."

"True, but I can't believe I did that. I am really sorry, Rebecca."

I was left speechless by his sincerity.

Jake continued, "Why don't you come over here and let me make it up to you."

"Tonight?!"

"Yeah, right now. Come over. Let me make it up to you."

I felt like shit, and I had to get up in eight hours. I had no intention of leaving my apartment, not even for Jake Thompson.

"You'll make it up to me, huh? And how do you intend to do that? Tell me."

Jake proceeded with an X-rated description of what he'd do for me, to me, with me, you name it. That boy had a voice, and a style, that could put any girl into submission. I was back on the floor, playing with the telephone cord, but it didn't take long for me to tell him to shut up.

"Jake, I can't come over tonight."

"Why not?" He sounded shocked and disappointed. I had never heard him like that before. He was playing my role.

"I have one week left of summer quarter. I need to sleep well, and if you keep talking like that, I'm not gonna be able to get you out of my head, and I'll be up all night."

"Well, then come on over!"

"Fuck you, Jake." I gently pounded on my pillow along with every word. "Fuck you."

"Why, Gould? What's the matter?"

"The matter, *Jake*, is that you're telling me to come over so that we can finally release five years' worth of sexual tension, and

I'm *not* gonna come over tonight, and next time we talk, you'll probably tell me that I missed my 'opportunity' because you're 'temperamental,' and that's what happened during winter break and earlier this summer, and you and I both know that we're all talk anyway."

"It's not like that this time, Rebecca. I'm not gonna change my mind and let you down again. Just come over."

"Jake! I told you: not tonight. If you're for real, then you'll quit trying to get me to come over tonight. You'll call me tomorrow, we'll get together at the end of the week, and you'll prove me wrong."

"It's a deal, Rebecca."

"Fine," I sighed and looked at the clock.

It was time for bed, but Jake read my mind before I could make my get-away.

"Well, Gould, it's eleven o'clock. I've gotta sleep. You've gotta sleep—"

"Yeah, yeah. I know."

"But I'll call you tomorrow night after I've talked to my boss, okay?"

"Okay. Good night, Jake."

"Good night, Rebecca."

We never did take that road trip. But it wasn't long after that phone call that we finally had our one night of passion—well, if you could even call it that. We had sex. Didn't feel very passionate. I didn't cum. I mean, it was okay, but mostly it felt surreal. After so many years of anticipation, the big event was anticlimactic, literally and figuratively.

So you'd think I'd have stopped fantasizing about Jake in order to get myself off, right?

Right, for a while. But not for long. My body was so trained to respond to the fantasy of him that I convinced myself that if we'd just had one more night together, one more chance, it would have been amazing. I had to hold onto the fantasy—up until I met Brian. I actually did stop thinking about Jake for the most part, until I got tired of not having orgasms when having sex with my new boyfriend and soon-to-be-fiancé, soon-to-be ex-husband.

I rationalized that the fantasy helped me break the ice or something, and from then on I'd be able to cum without thinking of another man. I thought I could switch Jake out for Brian, my true love. And sometimes that was the case. But oftentimes, I still needed the fantasy to get off.

Looking back at it now, over ten years later, it's as if I were a completely different person. Now I am so dedicated to the truth, to reality and authenticity. The thought of thinking about one man while with another feels icky to me now. No shame if that's what floats *your* boat. But for me, I get off on being fully present.

Fully in truth. Fully embracing the reality of who I am with and what is happening. Even when I masturbate—yes, sometimes I do fantasize a little, but more often than not I cum while being fully aware of what it is I'm doing with myself, for myself. And the other day, while writing this, I did a little experiment: I tried thinking of Jake while masturbating.

Guess what? It didn't work. I'm grateful for all the times it brought me so much pleasure. But I'm even more grateful to be free of that trap. Free to experience massive amounts of pleasure and the full extent of sexual release by being fully present instead of escaping reality by thinking of something or someone who isn't even good for me. I'm grateful that I don't need another person, in reality or in fantasy, in order to cum. That is liberation. That is sexual freedom. And I know that I'll never be trapped again.

About the Author

Rebecca Clio Gould

www.rebeccacliogould.com
www.themultiorgasmicdiet.com

If you could give one piece of advice to your younger self about your orgasm, what would it be?

The advice I'd give to my younger self about orgasm is to not feel any pressure to have one when receiving oral sex, and to just enjoy what's happening without agenda. And if it's not enjoyable, make suggestions for what sort of touch would feel better.

If your orgasm had a voice, what would your orgasm say to you about the piece you wrote for this book?

My orgasm would say, "Woo hoo! Whether using fantasy or reality to get off, way to take control of your own pleasure!"

Anything else you would like to add about your story or the experience of writing it?

"The Fantasy Trap" is part of a longer story that might someday be a book. Although I share some very personal, intimate things in my book The Multi-Orgasmic Diet, this story felt edgy to me in terms of making such a personal story public. It also felt liberating and inspiring, as most edge-pushing endeavors do.

As for my story, "The Multi-Orgasmic Diet," it's slightly adapted from the piece I published through Elephant Journal. In that story, masturbation is just one option out of over 80 practices on the diet menu, and my masturbation diet was definitely a fun experiment!

I hope both of these contributions help readers brush away shame and guilt and open up to more pleasure in their lives.

Chapter 8
MY GOD, MY ELVIS
By Dawna Phillips

He really was a god. Yes, they called him the King, but he was far more than that. He was a god to me. I don't remember when I fell in love with Elvis. It had to be the moment I first saw him, probably on-screen at a movie theater. Elvis was the most beautiful man I had ever seen. I found it difficult to believe such a perfect human could have been created, and there he was on the very large screen in front of me, just a bit out of reach. I guess you can't touch a god.

Elvis was an only child. I grew up in a large family of half- and step-siblings. Altogether there were twelve. I am the middle child of the seven siblings I grew up with, six girls and one boy. I was the fourth oldest and fourth youngest. I had two older sisters and a brother who was born ten and a half months before I came along. He weighed in at twelve pounds. Since he was born at home with a midwife, they took him to the local store to weigh him on the meat scale. He was a big baby. Ten and a half months later, I arrived and was Mom's smallest, at seven pounds one ounce. A year and five days after my arrival, a sister came along. A year and four days after her, another sister popped out. A few years following her birth, enter stepfather and another sister.

I was born in Hudson Bay, Saskatchewan, Canada, the nearest town to Armit, where we lived. Armit is a small lumber town in northern Saskatchewan. Even though we left Armit when I was three, I remember the house we lived in. In front of the house there were wild rose bushes. As a little girl I would pluck off a pink rosebud and pretend to use it for lipstick. We didn't have much to play with except the junk scattered around the yard, so our imaginations were our biggest toys. One of the things that littered the yard was a small cast-iron frying pan. As the story goes, my biological father, or my bio-dad, was in a wheel chair due to polio by this time and was looking out the window. He saw me standing in one spot, holding the frying pan and staring at him. He told my mother he believed I looked as if I were taking aim and suggested she get out there before I threw it. Apparently she looked at me through the window, but before she could get out the door the frying pan went flying through the glass at bio-father. I was told that he beat her from time to time, and although I don't remember the beatings, I think toddler Dawna may have decided to punish him for hurting her mother. This was 1954, and since it was summer I would have been about two and a half. That same year, Elvis was auditioning with a house band in Memphis and was told he'd never make it as a singer.

Four years later, as Elvis was awarded his first gold album and driving around in a pink Cadillac, my mother loaded all six of us in a car with this strange man who was to become our stepfather. I don't think any of us had ever been in a car before. We went to Calder, Saskatchewan very briefly before moving to Kamsack. While Elvis was releasing my favorite of his movies, *Jailhouse*

Rock, we moved into a house just across the street from the police station. The rent was fifty dollars a month. Ironically, maybe I was entering my own prison.

One day when I was six I was on the sidewalk playing hopscotch alone. An old man came by and was friendly to me. He asked me if I wanted a dime. Of course I did! A dime could buy lots of things back then. He said I had to give him a kiss for that dime. Seemed simple enough. My mother was watching this out the window, came out, and lit into this old pervert with a tirade. This sticks in my head because the rest of the family, instigated by the stepfather, decided that teasing me that this old man was my boyfriend was funny. I was so embarrassed. While I was being hit on by an old fart on the sidewalk in front of my house, Elvis was being drafted into the army and lost his signature pompadour. I wonder what I lost that day.

From the time my mother left bio-father until I was ten, I had the same dream every night. This dream took place in that first house, which may be the reason I remember a lot of details about that house. In the dream there was a large hole in the middle of the living room floor, and if you fell down into that hole, there were people there who kept you and fattened you up. These people talked a lot. You then shed your skin and were tossed back onto the main floor. Out the front door was a man who would flick his tongue at you and catch you on a string and keep you with him until you could get away. Out the front door was always winter. Out the back door was a man who would flick his fingers out, kind of like Spiderman does with his web, and catch you on a string and keep you there until you could escape. Out the back door was always muddy. Upstairs was another man who did the finger flick, only with the hand the other way around, knuckles up, and he caught you on a string and kept you until you could get away. I don't remember ever getting away or being caught. I do remember falling into the hole in the living room. Being thrown up with new skin wasn't frightening at all. I had this dream every night, and every night I would wake up and stay awake for who knows how long, but for what seemed like an eternity. I would listen and think I heard people living in our house while we slept. One night when I was ten, I slept the night through and never had the dream again.

My favorite dreams after that were my dreams of Elvis. There were many throughout the years. Growing up I went to every one of his movies and would usually sit through them twice. The movie cost fifteen cents, twenty-five if it was a double feature. I was sure I was going to marry Elvis someday.

We had an outhouse for a while until the landlady put in running water. Before that, the mother would put a red rag on a stick in the alley so that the waterman knew we needed water. He would fill up a large barrel in the back porch with water that would last us all week. We had a wood stove at that time, too, and the mother would have to heat water once a week and fill a large tub, which we all had to bathe in.

The stepfather was a truck driver back in the days when truck drivers didn't make much money. He would be away for days at a time. One time when he came home and asked how we were while he was gone, my mother must have said not-too-happy things about us. He lined us up in front of him and was going to give us a lickin' one at a time, you know, over the knee, bare-bottomed, with a switch. Brilliant six-year-old Dawna decided to stand in the middle of the line so she wouldn't be first, not knowing which end he was going to start at. Well, he started in the middle with me.

We all played outside a great deal. When we were underfoot, mother would always say, "Go outside and play." The stepfather on the other hand would always make it sound like playing was not a good thing, and we should be doing something useful all the time. It was in the fall, and we were improvising with what we had to play with. I decided to pretend to play golf with the blunt end of an ax and a rock. When I went to hit the rock, my little half-sister fell or was pushed in front of the ax, and I hit her in the mouth, knocking her front baby teeth up into her gums. All hell broke loose. My stepfather was on the road. My mother kept saying to me, "Just wait until your father (we were told to call him that) gets home." This baby sister being his only blood daughter made her his favorite, so we thought. I think it was about three days, but for me it was an eternity. In the time it took him to return home I went through pure hell. I considered running away, but to where? I considered suicide so as not to get the lickin', but how could I do that so it wouldn't hurt, too? When he did finally arrive home I was expecting maybe to be beaten to death. But after hearing the story and I guess seeing the fear on my face, or for whatever reason, he said, "I think she has suffered enough" and didn't touch me—at least not then. If I could exchange that beating for what was to follow, I would in a heartbeat.

In 1964, as my Elvis was in the throes of being dethroned as King of the Charts by the Beatles, I lost an innocence I would never get back. Our stepfather, whom we were told was our savior, thought that feeling us up was funny, something to joke about. He would come downstairs after feeling up my brother and tell everyone that he had a morning hard-on. He would stick his hand in our pants and smell his fingers afterward. When we girls started getting, or sprouting he called it, boobs, he was very verbal when pointing it out or groping us at every chance he got. We had to fight him off whenever he caught us alone to keep his hands out of our pants. One time when I was twelve I was alone in the bedroom. He came in and started to fondle me. I fought him off as much as I could until he finally had my pants down. He told me I was a freak—my genitals were all wrong, and I was turning into a man.

I was twelve, and my inner labia were new to me, and they were all poofy. He said I was growing balls. When he said this I panicked. Those words and his vigilant staring at me, watching for signs of the transformation to a man, had me thinking I was a freak for many years. He would announce to everyone that I was growing an Adam's apple. I sat in school touching my neck and feeling for an Adam's apple. I pushed tongue up against the roof of my mouth to suck in any hint of a bulging bone. I was skinny, so every bone showed anyway. I would stare at myself in the mirror, looking for signs of something male to happen, like facial hair. I thought my eyebrows were going to be a unibrow because I was turning into a man. I lay in bed at night touching myself and rubbing the labia minora, hoping I could rub them off because my stepfather had me convinced they were growing into balls.

A few years earlier a friend had showed me how to masturbate the clitoris, although I didn't know that is what it was called at the time, and she called it fucking yourself. Of course this felt good, so I did it from time to time, feeling pleasure and guilt at the same time. I even thought that maybe doing this is what caused the gender confusion. After the stepfather's invasion I thought that thing was going to grow into a penis. I believed a woman should just have the two lips and a hole. That should be it. Not all this other stuff that suddenly appeared. I don't even know if it was sudden, I just didn't notice it before it was pointed out by a pervert who should have known better and shouldn't have been poking around in the first place.

The stepfather would make lurid comments to all of us. He would say, "Why do you need an education to change diapers?" Because we were mostly girls, we were told we were all whores who had no control where sex was involved.

Time went on with me truly believing I was a freak of nature. I had crushes, but would every boy who looked at me see what I really was? How would I ever have sex with a man? How could I ever let anyone look at me "down there"? I never really dated anyone. I had my first kiss when I was fifteen. My second oldest sister came and got me one night when she and her boyfriend had another guy who needed a date. I am sure my sister was doing the hokey pokey in the front seat, and this guy thought I should be doing it with him in the back, but that wasn't going to happen. That would have been weird—my first kiss and my first boink all on the same night as my "first date"!

It was the spring of 1967. I went to the movies with my sister. We saw *The Greatest Story Ever Told*. I cried. When we arrived home and walked into the living room, there sitting on the couch was a man who I thought looked just like Jesus in the movie. He was the son of the stepfather who hadn't seen his father since he was five. He lived 2,000 miles away in Ontario. When he was twenty he decided to leave Ontario in search of his father. I fell immediately in love with Larry as only a fifteen-year-old can, but believing nothing could happen since he was my "brother," albeit a step one with no blood ties. Also there was the problem of me turning into a male. He had brought three other rather good-looking guys with him. With a house full of teenage girls they, I am sure, thought they had hit the jackpot. I think we did, too. I started dating one of them named Harry. One night during a make-out session all of a sudden it was in *oweeee!* and that was the end of my virginity. As I was accidentally losing my virginity, my Elvis was marrying someone else.

Larry and these friends left after a few months. I spent the next few months pining away for him. Before he left, though, I had drank a bit more wine than was good for me one night and professed my love for him. Everyone laughed about it, and that should have been the end of that.

The next spring Larry returned. One day he asked me to go for a drive with him for some made-up reason. I did, and eventually we did the hokey pokey. We had been sneaking around for a few months because we figured we shouldn't be dating because of the step-sibling issue. That fall, when I found out I was pregnant, I was in total panic. First, I had this freak thing still happening. I actually thought that because I was a freak I was safe from getting pregnant. But there I was, a frightened, pregnant little girl with a freak complex. I really wanted to undo this, but abortion was not even on the table. Larry finally told our parents and, believe it or not, they were thrilled that their kids were getting married to each other. Marriage was inevitable and welcomed even though we didn't have a pot to piss in. We borrowed $50 to get married. But I was marrying the man I was in love with as much as you can be in love at sixteen. He wasn't Elvis, but Elvis had married someone else. And his daughter was born that March.

Larry had actually beaten the crap out of me before we got married, but you know the thought—*I am sure after we are married that won't ever happen because we are in love.* He was good-looking, and at sixteen, that was love to me. The parents had their kids marrying each other and a blood grandchild for both of them.

Here is a weird part of this—I want to say drama, but the right word is trauma—I went to the doctor at about three months into the pregnancy. We all knew I was pregnant, but the doctor didn't give me an internal examination then or at all during the entire pregnancy. I was so terrified of that examination because I just knew he was going to laugh when he saw my genitals because I was a freak. I knew my husband wasn't the brightest crayon in the box, so I thought he just didn't know I was a freak. But surely a doctor would know. My breasts started leaking at three months, and my mother told me that wasn't normal, and that only fueled the freak fire. During the pregnancy my baby had the hiccups. My imagination took me to the far reaches of freak zone, and I just knew if I were a freak, I must be having a freak baby. Ultrasound would have fixed that, but in 1969 it was unheard of.

I was due the beginning of April. It was the end of the second week in April, and my doctor decided to go on holidays. In came a new doc from Winnipeg for my next examination. Of course he knew I was overdue and wanted to give me an internal examination. I panicked. How could I get out of this? I undressed and got on the examination table, shaking uncontrollably. I think he just thought I was cold and put another sheet over me. He asked me to spread my knees and I started to cry and couldn't, and I couldn't tell him why. Finally he brought in a couple of nurses to hold my knees apart so he could examine me. I think they chalked my reactions up to my age and being shy. He didn't laugh or jump back in shock. In the back of my terrified mind, I thought he and the nurses were just being nice so as not to hurt my feelings. That night I started having pains, and Larry took me to the hospital. This was small-town Saskatchewan, so small-town hospital. Of course, as soon as I get there they had to examine me. Same thing happened, I held my knees so locked together they hurt. The nurses, once again, came in to assist, probably again chalking it up to my age. They probably wondered how I managed to get pregnant in the first place. When they examined me again, no one laughed or looked shocked. The pains went on the same until the next morning. At noon they gave me a labor-inducing shot. By this time I thought every person in Kamsack had had a peek at my vagina, and no one said anything or looked shocked or laughed, but I believed they were probably somewhere discussing the freak about to give birth. At 6:35 p.m. a gorgeous nine-pound four-ounce baby boy popped out, with the help of forceps. They showed him to me and I cried. He was the most beautiful baby ever born on this planet, with all his human bits in the right places. His skin was clear and the prettiest shade of pink. He looked a month old already. You'd think that would have rested my freak issue forever. It didn't.

I went on with my married life. Sex was basic sex when he wanted it. I had another son in 1971, still believing I was a freak and no one would tell me for sure. Everyone was just being nice. Then one day my husband brought home a girly magazine. I reluctantly paged through it when he was at work. I am not sure why I thought I needed to be sneaky about looking in the magazine. Guiltily turning the pages, I paused in shock and disbelief. Right there on the page in front of me was a woman casually sitting spread-eagle, displaying her vagina for all to view.

I was totally shocked. It was no different than mine. I was normal. All those years with all those fears of someone outing me as a freak were for nothing. I asked my husband if I was the same as the other women he had been with. He said more or less. It never, ever occurred to me to ask him that question sooner. I guess I didn't want to point out any imperfections or freaky anomalies he hadn't noticed. We then talked more about sex and started to do different things. I wasn't as embarrassed anymore. I finally had an oral sex orgasm and never looked back. While Elvis was divorcing Priscilla, I discovered that I was perfectly normal.

When I was pregnant with my last son I was sure I was going to have a girl. All my friends who had had girls gave me their girl infant clothes. Everyone was convinced I was having a girl. I was really excited when I went into labor. I was going to meet my little girl, Misty Dawn. I already had two sons, and this little girl would complete the family. She would have two older brothers to look after her. When the baby arrived weighing in at nine pounds three ounces, they told me it was another boy. I really wanted to cry, but when they showed him to me I saw the cutest little boy with a giant melon-head and long black hair. They asked me what his name was, and I hadn't chosen a boy's name. I didn't want to admit this, so I said the first name that came to mind. I had been watching the movie *Tickle Me* the night before. Elvis's name in the movie was Lonny, so I said Lonny. I maybe could have changed my mind, but every time they brought him to me they would say, "Here's Lonny."

After Lonny was born, I looked at Larry and wondered why I'd ever married him. He was abusive at times and put me in the hospital once with a big gash on my face. He had hit me with the coffee table. He was a bricklayer by trade, and in the harsh Ontario winters there wasn't a lot of bricklaying to be done. One winter when Lonny was two Larry decided to go work in a bar as a bartender. He was still fairly attractive, and he realized that there were women coming on to him. He never cheated on me, but as a bartender he wanted to, so he came home one day and said to me, "How about we split up for a while?" I couldn't believe my ears. I said yes without hesitation. I'd thought of leaving many times, but I believed I couldn't leave and live. I was sure he would kill me. He had guns. I was thrilled when he suggested leaving. This was in April. About two weeks after he left I panicked and begged him to come back. I had never been on my own before, let alone with three small boys. The best thing he ever did for me was to say no.

I was working in a yarn factory as a reeler at the time. I knew I didn't want to do that for the rest of my life. That year I turned twenty-five on January 6th, and on February 2nd I got my driver's license. I remember the date because it was Groundhog Day, and there were ten-foot snow banks on the corners, so I couldn't follow all the driving rules exactly. Larry bought me a '72 Oldsmobile, and we moved to an even smaller town. The factory I worked in was about ten miles from where we lived so the car and my license were necessary. I really can't imagine what my life would be like now if I hadn't gotten my driver's license when I did.

I phoned his mother to tell her of the split. She lived in Kitchener, the nearest city, which was about fifty miles away. She was very supportive and eventually helped me find an apartment in the city. I applied for assistance, enrolled in business college that fall, found a sitter, and was on my way. I stayed working at the yarn factory until I had to be in the city for college in September. The ex even helped me move my furniture to the apartment.

August 16, 1977. It was the saddest day of my life. I was still in the smallest town in Southern Ontario, getting ready to move to the city. After work every day I shed my work clothes and pop into my bikini and walk the two blocks to the store to buy what I needed to make supper that night. I would put what I bought on store credit until payday. Sue, the owner, and I became very good friends, and I would spend the time catching up on the local gossip and sharing stories. That day I walked down the street in my homemade blue polka-dot bikini, enjoying the sun on my skin and wondering what the future held. When I got to the store, Sue didn't greet me with her usual "happy-to-see-you" smile.

"What is wrong?" I asked, becoming concerned.

"I have some really sad news for you, Dawna." she said, her eyes tearing.

"What is it?" I thought something had happened to her husband and was ready to comfort her.

"Elvis is dead." She came to give me a hug. She knew my passion for Elvis only too well. My fantasy world fell apart at that moment. I was devastated.

I don't remember buying anything or walking home. How could this happen? Not my Elvis. I thought he would wait for me, and just when I was available he went and died.

The last time I saw Elvis was in a dream. He came to me regularly in my dreams. He hasn't been around for a few years. I am so grateful for the time we did have together, albeit in another dimension. I wonder, where is he now? Maybe like a true god, he has ascended, yet again, just beyond my reach.

About the Author

Dawna Phillips

What did you want to be when you were eight years old?

A ballerina (I wanted to dance), a model (I wanted pretty clothes), a princess (I wanted magic and the prince and the clothes and the castle . . . that list goes on forever).

If you could give advice to your younger self about your orgasm (or your body), what would it be?

Holy crap, where do I start? This question makes me cry. What would I tell little Dawna? I would tell her she is not a freak. I would tell her to love her body, that she and her body are beautiful and there is nothing wrong with her body or her. I would hug her. I would tell her she is not dirty and smelly. I would sit and talk to her about her feelings and the changes going on in her body and explain that everything that is happening, all the changes, are normal and to love the changes. I would tell her not to be ashamed of who she is and what she wears. I would tell her to speak up and tell someone how she feels. I would be there for her. Most of all I would give her that girly magazine when she was considering mutilating herself and encourage her to try and not be a freak.

If your orgasm had a voice, what would it say to you about the piece you wrote for this book?

It would say, Dawna you are very brave to tell your story. Your voice is a gift you have to help you heal us, to join us and make us one. There is no shame, no guilt and nothing to be afraid of. I am here, I am yours, own me and love me. Let me loose and let me fly.

Chapter 9
LOSING MY ORGASM, FINDING MYSELF
By Tara Rachyl Robertson

Things that have been said to me about me in regards to my sensuality include:

"Why won't you just put out . . . like all the other girls?!?"

Age 14.

This query delivered by my second ever boyfriend, Reg, in the days that followed my first ever attendance to a prom. At 14, I was a freshman cheerleader in high school. Reg was 17, in his junior year at high school, and on the varsity football team. I don't remember having a chance to respond to his query before he asked for his class ring back, thus ending our high-school romance and effectively deflating my social standing amongst my peers at the Catholic high school we attended.

"Aren't you just a little sexpot??"

Age 16.

No, in fact, I was not. I was still a virgin, actually. This hypothesis was proffered to me by Mr. Cunegan, my social studies teacher in Grade 11 after lunch one day, in front of the entire class of students.

"Come on, baby. Why should we wait? We're getting married anyway."

Age 19.

This was certainly not my first experience at being pressured for intercourse, and I was no longer a virgin at this stage in my young life. But, this pressurer . . . well, this one, he was supposed to love and honour and cherish me. Arjay and I were engaged. We had attended the local church's youth group together, where we both seemingly espoused a belief in chastity as a way of right living. His father was a deacon, and our parents were so very approving of our pairing. We never married, but we did fall pregnant twice—the first ending in miscarriage later that same year, the second, two years later, resulting in the birth of a beautiful daughter whom I placed in an open adoption.

"Come with me . . . I want to taste you, and then you can taste me when I spill down your throat."

Age 23.

These words were spoken at the start of a first date with a man 16 years my senior.

"You know you're hot, right? We should hook up. It's not illegal ya know . . . it's just frowned upon."

Age 26.

This illicit suggestion floated to me by a distant male cousin as if the only thing blocking us from coupling were a question of the legalities.

"I'm going to turn you out!"

Age 27.

This particular comment thrown my way by Bruno, a corrections officer with an anger problem, a porn addiction, and a social calendar that revolved entirely around WWE's television programming.

As I reflect on this selection of just a handful of the explicit comments I have received about myself throughout my life, what stands out to me is that all these men have a common sense of entitlement to MY body. It seemingly mattered not if I was inclined in the same way towards them; it was enough that they wanted me. As I was recalling each encounter, I actually caught my own breath as I remembered another shocking comment I received. Age 29, my then-future-husband made this comment to me whilst returning home one night following our date: "I can have you whenever I want." I married him six months later.

Dane and I had been dating for maybe a month at the time of his assertion. We were quite the cosmopolitan, jet-setting couple. He was Australian, and I was an American studying at an Australian university. I lived in a plush, sub-penthouse apartment in the heart of Melbourne's inner suburbs, on the city's esteemed St Kilda Road and he lived 1500 kilometers away in Brisbane. One of us would have to hop on a plane and fly to other in order to "date." It was exciting and felt a bit glamorous. Dane was well-connected thanks to his career as a chef, and he knew all the best places to take me out in both cities.

On the particular evening Dane declared that he could "have [me] whenever [he] wanted," we had been out for a romantic walk and decadent meal at the in-demand restaurant Botanical. I recall two very strong emotions that night. The first, a feeling of floating as we walked hand-in-hand around Melbourne's much-lauded Royal Botanic Gardens. I remember looking in his eyes as we slowly strolled together, thinking, *Is this what being 'in love' feels like? Am I falling in love with this guy right now?* The second, a rather strong feeling of apprehension as he made his declaration, smacked my bum, and pulled me firmly into him, kissing me aggressively on the street just outside my unit. I was fearful about what was going to transpire once we were alone in the privacy of my apartment. But I stayed quiet.

Though we were only newly dating and still barely known to each other, this was already the second time in our relationship I had actively silenced my own intuitive voice about Dane. Silencing my own voice, my own desires became the norm with Dane.

I am a woman who has never shied away from pursuing a sexual exploit. Thanks to my rather traumatic forays into love and motherhood with Arjay at 19 and again at 22, I learned early on in adult life to escape emotional turmoil by throwing myself into sexual escapades. Why feel or even risk emotional pain when I could soar on orgasmic pleasure, walk away when it was all over and move on to the next high? And there was always a next high to be found. I knew exactly how to use a man's body to reach that euphoric state. I was brazen and unafraid of telling someone precisely how I wanted to be fucked in any given escapade. Throughout my twenties, I proudly embraced lyric from the song "Independent Women" by Destiny's Child: "When it's all over, please get up and leave." Queen of the one-night stand, me.

By the time I reached 29, I had long since stopped counting my lovers because 1) my body, my rules and 2) as long as I was safe and protected and not causing harm to another, what the hell difference did a number make? So, when I married Dane in 2007, I made the very decided choice to "settle down" and be a "good girl" once and for all. I imagined it must have pleased my family, and especially my mother, that I finally found a man to get serious with. I put aside my promiscuous ways and agreed to "forever" and "only" and "faithful." And I meant it, every word in my vows. But, something about my new husband never set well with me—he would never, ever, ever allow me to speak of my past. It was if that part of me never existed.

I thought marriage meant that sexual union would actually mean something. The existential bliss promised from two becoming one would be mine to know at long last. Only, for me, it never felt like that. To me, it wasn't different—it was the same as nearly any other sexual encounter I had known . . . only with the same person day after day.

In 2015, Dane advised me in the car one afternoon that he "didn't want to do this anymore." There was no discussion, no joint agreement or decision on the matter. I was simply informed by my husband of eight years that he was done with being married to me. The tone and demeanour of his announcement was not at all dissimilar to his assertion during our dating days that he could "have [me] whenever [he] wanted." And since Dane got what Dane wanted when he wanted it during our marriage, that was that. Marriage over.

His announcement came in the midst of me having a series of significant health challenges over the better part of two years, including a stroke at age 35 and nine weeks in the hospital as an in-patient to recover from a shattered ankle. Under Australian law, it takes at least 12 months to have a divorce granted. Because of another setback in my health, it was 15 months before I filed. Not surprisingly, I was left to be the one who had to figure out the technicalities of dissolving our union; doing so was not on his "list of priorities" for moving on with his life.

By the time a judge granted our divorce, I had returned to my hometown of Indianapolis. Returning home was a symbolic and literal return to myself after more than a decade away. In the month immediately following the receipt of my divorce decree, I was surprised to find myself deeply blushing during a conversation with colleagues at my job in a medical office about the anatomy and physiology of the female orgasm. After treating a pregnant patient, Dr. Yemmik, the physician staffing the clinic, was discussing in great detail the wonder it is that a woman ever successfully becomes pregnant because of the angle of the vagina and cervix and what has to physically happen in a woman's body for fertilization to occur. Dr. Yemmik explained in particular detail the aspects involving the cervix opening and "scooping" up the semen.

At this particular point of the discussion, my colleagues noted, with great amusement, my face rapidly flushing to a scarlet shade as I had an immediate and profound insight. After 39 years of inhabiting this female body, having been pregnant three times, I had only just learned exactly how my own anatomy is designed and works for ultimate pleasure. This led me to the incredulous realization that I could actively recall only a single orgasm experienced with my husband. Through this lesson in intimate anatomy, I also learned exactly how a woman becomes pregnant. The memory of that particular orgasm was triggered precisely because it had led to us becoming pregnant just three months into our marriage, a pregnancy I insisted we end because every inch of my psyche was utterly resistant to the idea of offspring with Dane. Weeks of rising panic rushed over me like waves, the ever-increasing weight of dread as the pregnancy progressed threatened to destroy my mental health. Turns out, I didn't always silence my intuitive voice. I listened when it screamed at me. I could find my voice when pushed to the edge.

That workplace conversation became a catalyst for my reflection on my marriage and how I participated in it. I knew and had admitted to a few close girlfriends how physically dissatisfied I had become in my marriage. I had lamented Dane's lack of effort or ingenuity in our lovemaking. It had become fast, detached, and functional. He only seemed interested in slamming himself into me whenever he wanted a release. He was completely unconcerned with my satisfaction and insistent that I be willing, ready, and able at his beck and call. I had so completely disconnected from the brazen woman who readily spoke up for my own pleasure and instead had simply become his living love doll. At one point, I had even taken myself off to the doctor to discuss whether there was something physically wrong with me as I could no longer ignore my considerable disinterest in sex. I wondered, was I having some abnormal fluctuation in hormone levels as I neared 40? I had always enjoyed a healthy sexual appetite. My doctor's advice? That I schedule time in every week for sex. "Sometimes, you just have to treat it as any other wifely chore that needs doing," he counselled.

My reflections on my participation in my marriage revealed to me how much I actively ignored the intuitive language of my own body as it pertained to my own pleasure. It seemed to me that in realising how long I had been without orgasm in my life, I came to realise how long I had been without feeling in my life generally. I had merely been going along, participating in it in the ways that I perceived others expected of me. And in doing so, I had so completely disconnected from my own pleasure that I wasn't even aware that it was missing for the better part of a decade. What an absolute tragedy.

But, this tragic realisation was my catharsis. Without it, I would not have fully returned to myself. Without it, I would not have had the opportunity to reflect on my what sensual life was before marriage and what it became during marriage. Without it, I would not have been prompted to enquire of myself how I desire it to be following on from marriage. I now can articulate what sensual pleasure has meant in my past. And I am so much clearer on the exact way I wish to experience sensual pleasure in my life going forward.

To some, my sensual past will surely look have looked totally Super Whore. So be it. To me, it was it was the not only a means of self-preservation from the pain of my decisions born of naiveté, but equally a way to discover my own brazen and cavalier approach to life itself. Without becoming the woman who actively sought out orgasmic experiences as a means of escape, I would not have become the woman who was confident enough to take on solo travel adventures across the country and the world, who then became the woman self-assured enough to pack up her life and migrate to the other side of the planet in just six short months once she finally figured out what she wanted to be when she grew up. And I damn sure wouldn't be the tenacious, persevering woman I am today had I not learned to be bold earlier in my life.

So, now, I'm clear: I want to be opened to the cosmos through my sensual life. I want to find that place of sensual union that is not born of sex as a connection, but rather as a sacred extension of connection. I want only the devotional kind of deep sexy found in the mutual honouring of each other's divine gifts and activation of each other's heart centres.

From here, the sensual woman I choose to be post-marriage will only move forward towards my heart's desire. No longer will

I allow my sensuality to be treated as anything other than absolutely sacrosanct and deserving of reverence. I refuse to allow myself to disconnect from my desire for pleasure as I choose to define it in my life. Instead of simply saying "my body, my rules" I hereby embrace "my life, my rules." Those who choose not to regard them will be asked to leave. From here, the me that I choose to be post-marriage is only ever an active, connected participant in my life and my pleasure.

About the Author

Tara Rachyl Robertson

What did you want to be when you were eight years old?

A ballet dancer. Dancing is what I most remember loving as child. It actually took me until I was 27 before I figured out what I "wanted to be when I grow up." It took another 13 years beyond that to have a clear understanding of what my life purpose is.

If you could give one piece of advice to your younger self about your orgasm, what would it be?

Your enjoyment of sex IS SO IMPORTANT. It's as important as any partner's enjoyment. DO NOT sacrifice yourself for the sake of him. You are not simply there for his pleasure / enjoyment. You are there for yourself, as well. For god(dess)'s sake, if what's happening is not doing it for you, SPEAK UP FOR YOURSELF.

If your orgasm had a voice, what would your orgasm say to you about the piece you wrote for this book?

It's about damn time, woman!

Anything else you would like to add about your story or the experience of writing it?

Getting through recounting my life viewed through this particular lens was equal parts harder than I thought it would be and easier than I thought it would be. It was all parts therapy I didn't consciously know I needed. It gave me answers I'd loosely been seeking for myself outside of myself. Participating in Betsy Blankenbaker's work was instinctual to me because when I first encountered it, I had an immediate longing to have encountered its wisdom much, much earlier in my life. I feel privileged to be a part of keeping this conversation open for women. I feel blessed to be part of a group of sisters with shared experience and, now, a shared voice.

Chapter 10

CLEANING UP

By Erika Brooke

I remember one evening, the bathtub was filled with warm water, and bubbles formed, as he helped me undress. I got into the bathtub and began playing excitedly with the bubbles. I made a Santa beard on my face and giggled while saying, "Ho, Ho, Ho." He climbed in after me, totally naked, and the bubbles quickly surrounded him, too. He placed a washcloth over his thing that stuck out from his middle.

"Do you want to play?" he said. "We are going to play Snake in the Grass, which means you have to find the snake and tag it."

I was confused as to whether the grass was the bubbles or all that weird hair around what I guessed was the snake . . . attached to his middle . . . that I did not have. I thought something must be wrong with me. Playing Snake in the Grass is the earliest memory I have of my father. I was three.

Throughout my earliest years, birth to around age three, we moved around a lot, but the house I remembered most during that time was the one where the incident with my dad occurred. I have a few very fond memories there despite my young age and the bathtub game. One such memory is sneaking Oreo® cookies to the porch and licking the creamy middle out only to throw the cookie portion into the bushes to destroy the evidence. Also, the mice in that old farm-ish house with a gorgeous wood staircase must have been prevalent because my mom would tease us and say, "That's what's in the quiche!" Mouse quiche or not, it was delicious. Then again, most of my mom's cooking tasted awesome.

At night, when I slept in my parents' bed, I lay close to the edge of the bed in order to be as far away from my dad as possible. Just as I dozed off, I would awaken to visions of small skeletons and black smoke rising up towards me.

Mom and Dad divorced when I was three, so my dad, sister, brother, and I moved in with my dad's parents. I spent the next few years attached to my Grandma Carmen. I followed her everywhere, helping with what seemed to be non-stop chores while my brother, Joe, and sister, Michelle, went to school. She called me her "gopher." I assumed she meant a cute, rodent-like animal because I was small and full of energy, but eventually she explained that she meant "go for" as in go get this or go get that . . . "go for" this, "go for" that, which made way more sense! Despite their household being strict and stiflingly religious and my grandpa, who was a pastor, intermittently playing the piano as loudly as possible while he bellowed out any old hymn on his heart, I felt loved and safe.

We moved about an hour away at the beginning of second grade. I hated leaving my Grandma Carmen . . . she was my safe place. And soon after we moved, Michelle moved in with my mom and stepdad, which left another hole in my heart and simultaneously removed female companionship of any kind.

My brother and I took care of each other because my dad was not home often. I did the laundry and tried making dinner while Joe, who was six years older, struggled with his algebra. I found out later he also struggled with alcohol. I knew he would sneak beers, and I found empty cans hidden all over his room when I gathered his laundry, but I was too young to know the implications. At one point my mom tried getting help for him, but she got overruled by the men in the family. Finally, when I was nine years old and halfway through third grade, I got to move in with my mom, stepdad, and sister. I hated to leave Joe, but I wanted my mom. I desperately wanted to be nurtured again like Grandma Carmen had done.

I started at a new school. I played volleyball and basketball, made nearly straight A's in gifted classes, but I also drank, had sex with my boyfriends and smoked pot on occasion. I started my period when I was nine, so by thirteen it felt past due to begin exploring my sexuality further. I did not realize women were supposed to enjoy sex. In fact, when I would get wet while making out with a guy, I kept running to the bathroom to wipe it off. I figured that was wrong with me, too.

I loved the sense of accomplishment and validation I felt every time a guy's desire pulsated on me or in me, which immediately created intense shame and regret . . . only to repeat the cycle again.

The women in my family had big boobs and were valued for it. Not me. I had small boobs, so it was gratifying to be able to still make a guy cum! I felt desired while silently saying a big "fuck you" to my dad and stepdad for their incessant taunting about how small my breasts were.

I was smart and made good grades, so I was told, "One day you will make enough money to buy new ones."

I remember a goodbye hug after my dad visited me in college where he said, "You have absolutely no fucking chest at all, so why do you hug me like your tits are going to get in the way?"

Ironically, Michelle, who had big boobs was ridiculed, too. Her nickname was "Tits on a Stick" or "Shit for Brains" depending on whether math homework was involved. My sister has gone on to become a nurse in cardiac care . . . hardly "shit for brains" as she was called.

During Christmas break of my eighth-grade year, nine days after my fourteenth birthday, Joe called me about an hour prior to the time he was scheduled to pick me up for basketball practice, telling me he did not feel well and asking if I could find another ride. I hung up the phone, annoyed at him. While I was at practice, my brother put a bullet through his heart.

The weight of the blame I placed on myself crushed my soul. I assumed that between not asking my brother what didn't feel well and having sex, I had disappointed everyone. I believed that if I just loved others enough or was good enough (which I never felt I was, because I did not measure up to the "Christian" standards taught as truth) then I could "fix" or heal situations or people. I felt that I contributed to the pain my family was feeling because I did not fix it. I didn't even ask him why he couldn't pick me up. I kept on fucking, though, because whenever my boyfriend came I felt better for making him feel good. At that point, it really did not matter if God hated me because I hated me.

The summer after my brother killed himself, between eighth and ninth grade, I spent a lot of time with my best friend at the time, Renee, and her family. One night her dad allowed us to have a few adult beverages, and we talked a lot about Joe and how to continue living and coping with the loss. I trusted him, not only because he was a "cool" dad but because he seemed genuinely interested in the pain I carried in the aftermath of the tragic loss of my brother. Later that night, after Renee and her stepmom went to bed, her dad and I continued talking and drinking. I had a buzz but remained cognizant of our conversation and the subsequent placement of his dick in my mouth. We went from drinking to him asking me to lay my head in his lap while he played with my hair to him pulling his hard dick out and guiding my mouth closer and closer to it. He mentioned the stress release we could both experience if I sucked him. He grabbed my hair so he could better manipulate my head with one hand and his erection with the other, and I allowed him in my mouth.

A few months later I asked my parents to put me in counseling. The added shame of this incident put me in a self-proclaimed depression, and I did not want to take the same route my brother had chosen. I shared with my counselor about the night with Renee's dad, which abruptly ended our session and resulted in him telling my parents and the state. I WAS MORTIFIED, and I vowed to never share anything with anyone ever again. I felt betrayed, as he was the only person I told. I did not want anyone else to know. The public defender assigned to my case informed me that it did not bode well for me to get this guy convicted given that I was sexually active. Convicting him was not my goal—I'd just wanted to talk with someone about it—but I wondered what, then, was the point of the counselor reporting it? He knew of my sexual history and yet remained obligated to report it? Was the system also obligated to tell me this thirty-something-year-old man was less guilty for providing alcohol to me and then coercing his cock into my mouth where he blew his load, simply because I chose this activity with guys my own age? I remember after our evening on his couch, Renee's dad said to me, "Look at the mess you made." I had spit it out all over him. That entire debacle only reinforced my shame and disconnect from my body. I thought I was doing the right thing, using my voice and defending myself, only to be told I asked for it, essentially, and that it was my fault . . . apparently also my mess.

Today, at thirty-nine years old, I look back at these messes "of mine" filled with empathy and compassion for younger Erika. I have three children. Elizabeth is twelve, Ryan is fourteen, and Kathleen is fifteen. I want to teach my kids to love themselves early and that adults are responsible for their well-being, not the other way around.

As my children are now full swing in adolescence, I am grateful for the privilege of providing, protecting, nurturing, and supporting them as they navigate life and learn the sacredness of their bodies and their true inner worth as young women and men.

I realize that although I am outwardly very successful and healthy, I had not yet rescued little me and validated my own innocence in the experiences. Though I do make enough money to buy new boobs, after breastfeeding three healthy and tenacious babies, I feel no desire to alter my breasts. I want to set the example that our bodies are sacred and worthy of love and respect just as they are—and healthy sexuality is a gift arising from that knowing.

Finally, after all these years of carrying the shame, guilt, and disconnect with me, reliving the stories of loss, abandonment and loving sex, yet still more for the satisfaction I got from satisfying the man, I have come to believe time only assists in healing all wounds if I admit I am wounded. I entered relationships to heal in men what needed to be healed in me. Time had not healed me because I had not yet acknowledged I was wounded. I also realized it is normal to desire and want to be desired and that relationships ending in silent treatment could very well be because I go silent on myself when I am in them. I focused on meeting the man's needs and expectations, which I based on historical ideologies, instead of connecting with myself and receiving love.

I have always been good at loving others. Now it is time I demonstrate this love for my own self.

About the Author

Erika Brooke

On Healing:

Finally, at the age of thirty-eight, I sought grief counseling to assist with the simultaneous navigation of my second divorce, while caring for my best friend, who had moved in with us so we could care for her as she ended her long, grueling battle with cancer. The divorce finalized, and three months later I watched my soul sister die. During the time of this counseling, unexpected, graphic, disturbing, sexually explicit visions or "memories" surfaced. One image that played in my mind projector is having blister rashes on my vagina along with discomfort and pain in my early years. I am still not certain what the "memories" and the rashes signify, I only know my daughters never had this issue. Maybe I was allergic to the soap?

I am not exploring this because it feels good or to embarrass my family or to shame the dead. (My father died suddenly when I was twenty-two.) I am sharing it because it is part of my truth, and I reconciled it to feel whole and to understand how it has impacted my adult sexuality, choices in men, and ability to receive love. It has affected my idea of womanhood and gender roles and supposed attributes of a woman and a man. I am not blaming nor wallowing in victimhood. I believe releasing and healing traumatic memories will heal my physical body and create healthy space to dance in lasting love.

My ego and left-brain have done a fantastic job creating outward success as I sought to do, but in my inner being I still felt like something was wrong with me . . . I could not find lasting love. I still felt unwanted and alone. After two failed marriages, a dead best friend, and a series of promising relationships that failed to launch, I found myself in a Qoya class after visiting a shaman the week prior. I signed up because I wanted to tap into my feminine energy more. I wanted to rediscover my beauty and rescue little me, the one who settled for less and felt unworthy and repeatedly gave herself to men. The one who still would not settle for a subservient place in society just because I didn't have a dick or big boobs. I realized my idea of being a woman was further skewed because I was not like the women in my family. I had small boobs, they had big boobs. They have long-term marriages. I have two failed ones.

During the writing prompt at the end of a Qoya clas with Betsy Blankenbaker, I realized my inner child was still looking for a man to want me. To validate me. To cherish me as the woman I am. I realized that although I am outwardly very successful and healthy, I had stuffed my own essence and secretly still believed myself as unworthy of heroic love. I hushed my own voice, and I attracted men who, like me, are outwardly very attractive, financially successful, and intelligent, but deep inside something was broken. While I had deep compassion for them, I neglected to heal myself. I pacified myself with their attention and promises of a redeemed life and love together. We were all disconnected from our inner children via repression, denial, and substitution. I also realized, finally, that none of what happened to me was my fault, and my choices to numb the pain were "normal" coping mechanisms.

I am not dirty or worthless as a woman, and my breasts remain perky yet small even after nursing three babies. My brother killed himself for his own reasons, not because I failed to love him enough. I began releasing ownership of anything that violated my being. I truly forgave others and myself. So though I speak of some of the pain I experienced and how words spoken in our family impacted me, I currently have a close relationship with my mom and stepdad. We have survived a lot together, and they are first in line to help my kids and me whenever we need it.

Chapter 11

DEAR ELLA

By Betsy Blankenbaker

Me too. Those were the words that I heard over and over again from women who read my book, *Autobiography of an Orgasm*. The book is about the five years I researched orgasm as a way to heal.

Me too. I was molested as a child and was too scared to tell anyone.

Me too. I was a sexually curious teenager but felt taken advantage of by teenage boys who played with my body without asking permission.

Me too. I was raped in college, but because it was someone I knew, I didn't think it was rape so I stayed quiet.

Me too. I had sex with men, even with my husband, that wasn't satisfying.

Me too. I didn't think I could have an orgasm. It was easier just to fake it.

Me too. I thought something was wrong with me, and I was too embarrassed to talk to anyone about it.

Me too.

Many of the women asked for guidance on what to do next. How to reclaim and remember their body as both holy and as a vessel for joy? The clitoris has 8,000 nerve endings, more than twice the number in the tip of a penis. If women are wired to feel good, why are so many women walking around feeling bad—or even numb—in their bodies?

Two main things happened after my book came out. The first was that I stopped getting asked out on dates. Were men intimidated by my honesty? Or was it because they were afraid I would write about them? Maybe it was my age?

By the time I completed the book, I had healed my body from the sexual assault I experienced as a child and teenager and from a date rape as an adult. As my body healed, I felt myself coming to life at age fifty, a time when many women are being dismissed by our society. I had finally found my orgasm and was being told it was too late. In the media and in conversation with others, I was given the message I was too old to be valued for my body.

The second thing that happened was that I started receiving stories from women around the world, thanking me for writing the book. One of those letters came from a friend of a friend. Her name was Ella.

Dear Betsy,

Thank you for writing your book. Your courage has encouraged me to start the healing that I know I desperately need after rape in college and disconnection from my body. My mother was raped, too, and she never spoke about it.

How do you let go of so much shame? How do you enjoy a body that has brought you more pain than you care to admit?

—Ella

One of the most horrifying things Ella shared with me (and I'm sharing here with her permission) is that during the rape in college she was cut by one of the men raping her. He left visible scars all over her body. He told her she would never be wanted by another man.

When I met Ella, it was more than ten years after the rape. She was happily married to a wonderful man, and she had just given birth to her second child. Her smile and eyes twinkled. We sat chatting as she nursed her newborn with her other son cuddled next to her. She was glowing. Ella had a life that was fulfilling, and she was thoughtful about nurturing herself as much as she nurtured her children and husband. And she had a secret.

"Since the rape in college," she told me, "I have never had sex with my husband without my body being covered. I always leave a t-shirt or top covering my body. I don't want anyone to see the scars."

I know so many women, including myself at one time, who cover themselves due to scars on the inside or outside. Our bodies become a map of the history of our sex life. Our bodies also carry the history of our families and the collective wound women carry from so many of us being assaulted and not speaking up. But Ella had wounds that you could see, and she was careful to keep them covered, even from her husband.

I included Ella's letter and my response in *Autobiographies of Our Orgasms, Vol.* I and I'm offering my response again here.

Ella,

There is no one solution for everyone. We are all different, so it's really important to listen to your inner wisdom. I know at the start of my orgasm research, when I committed to the thirty days of stroking my clitoris just to feel whatever came up, I really had to pay attention to each stroke, listen to my body's feedback, and make the tiniest adjustments to try and feel even more. It was me becoming the expert on myself. I stopped judging myself and was instead just curious.

How do you get better at listening to your body? One thing that really helped me was taking Qoya classes. I'm not sure where you live, but you can check the website (www.loveqoya.com) for local classes and retreats and to see if it interests you. There are even free videos on the site. The classes are part dance and part yoga (no levels and no experience required). A Qoya class is designed to help you remember how your body likes to move by paying attention to the feeling in your body. I remember being a kid on the playground and only doing the things I loved during recess because they made me feel good. As a child, I wouldn't repeat a movement over and over again if it didn't feel good in my body. As adults, we shouldn't either. During every Qoya class, we spend one song shaking every part of our body. We shake as a way to reset on a cellular level and to move the stuck energy through us. It's using movement as medicine. Qoya was as important to me as the thirty days of stroking my clit to feel my orgasm again because it revealed to me how to listen to my body, and with each class, I feel like I liberate a little more of my authentic self. And the classes made it easier for me to listen to my body when I was doing the more intimate research to feel my orgasm.

I also recommend spending three to four minutes every morning and night giving yourself a massage. Put on a favorite song while you do it. I call it the *Water Blessing Massage Ritual*, because our bodies are over 70% water, and the self-massage is a way to imprint love on every part of your body. Remember when I wrote in *Autobiography of an Orgasm* about my nearly dead orchid coming back to life when I told it I loved it every day for thirty days? That is what this massage does—it sends the message of love to every cell. Imagine rubbing gratitude or love into every area of your body. Your cells will carry that message through the day or through the night as you sleep. It may sound like a corny thing to do—like telling a plant you love it—and it may be uncomfortable at first. Do it like your life depends on it because it does. Our vaginas and brains are connected, and when we cut off feeling from all the nerve endings in our genitals, we deny our brains the signals that nourish our bodies, stimulate our creativity and give us a sense of wellbeing. Try it for seven days, and then extend it to forty.

Commit to stroking your clitoris for fifteen minutes a day. Consider this, too, a sacred ritual, like a prayer honoring your body. I call this the *Sacred Orgasm Ritual*. Begin the ritual with a few minutes of sending deep breaths all the way into your womb and pelvis. This sends fresh, clean oxygen to the area and increases blood flow. Inhale into your womb and then exhale the breath through your genitals ten times. Then, inhale hum with every exhalation ten times. Next, trace ten circles around the outer lips of your vulva. Take it slowly, and notice whether you prefer a lighter touch or a firmer one. And then begin stroking your clit for fifteen minutes without any attachment to results. Your only goal is to feel whatever you are feeling and then make adjustments to see if you can feel even more.

I think many of us had mothers and grandmothers who experienced sexual trauma and never spoke about it or healed from it. Some of our great-great-grandmothers were even burned for it.

When we don't choose to heal, the shame and disillusionment get passed on to the next generation. We have to be braver than our mothers were, because we can't afford to pass this on to our daughters. And we can't afford to live less than fully in our bodies in this lifetime. If we do, we continue the cycle of abuse, except instead of the men who raped us or the boys who assaulted us in college, we become our own abusers by not choosing to heal and recover. It's a choice we make every day when we look in the mirror and see ourselves with love or see ourselves with judgment.

Releasing the shame and enjoying your body after the abuse you experienced requires you to be a tiny bit braver than you have been before. It's a choice. It's worth it. I know you can do it. I did.

—Betsy

About 18 months after I met Ella, I received a message from her.

"I had sex with my husband fully naked the other night," she wrote. "I know you know what a big deal that was for me."

Ella didn't need to write anymore. I knew it was a reclamation. I knew it was her remembering that a scar is a place that has healed.

I asked Ella if I could share her story so that we can all heal our scars both the ones seen and invisible.

Here is more of her story. Here is Ella being a little bit braver than before.

Betsy: How did the rape in college keep you from feeling safe/comfortable in your body?

Ella: Honestly, I don't think it really made a difference. I was constantly in a state of feeling uncomfortable in my own skin for as long as I can remember. I think that all it did was give me a definitive moment in time that I could point to and say, "See, this is why you are the way you are," but in reality, it didn't change all that much for me. This may sound crazy, but it the most honest way I know how to answer this question.

Did you tell anyone after it happened?

My behavior following my assault became incredibly harmful, and I was asked to leave my college dorm and subsequently kicked out of school, which meant my parents got involved and I had to move back home. I remember sitting at the kitchen table with my mom; she was screaming at me and demanding that I tell her what had happened. It was an extremely hostile environment (pretty common at our house). I felt like I was in a cop movie where the police are aggressively interrogating a criminal. When I finally said that I had been raped, my mother's first response was to smile. That image will be forever seared into my brain. My mother was a victim of a rape and perpetually used it as a tool to manipulate people. So really, I think she was deep-down happy. Not only did she have another tool to use to get people to feel sorry for her (which she did, "Poor me, I am so distraught—my daughter has been raped. Feel sorry for me!"), she had another tool with which to control me. She still to this day uses that as a way to keep me from growing and moving on with my life.

You mentioned your mom was raped. Did you ever discuss your experiences with each other?

Yes, but not in a healthy way. I feel like my understanding of sexual assault and rape had always been unique because that was my first introduction to sexuality. My mother would constantly talk about it and tell me horrifying details of cases on the news and of her own assault. I distinctly remember her telling me when I was eight years old that sometimes men don't rape you with their penises, they will use toothbrushes to do it. My eight-year-old brain did not know how to process that kind of information.

I guess that was her way of preparing me for life, but all it really did was plant deep seeds of distrust of sex, and that sex was a gross thing that bad men did to women who weren't careful. But as I write that, I have to say that at a certain point in my adolescence I became curious about rape in an unhealthy way. Kinda like, let's just get this rape thing over with so I can be done with it. I clearly just assumed that it was going to happen to me, considering that's all I heard about growing up.

Why do you think you were afraid to speak up?

I don't think I was afraid to speak up initially, but I eventually became afraid of what that meant for my life. The only other example was that of my mother, and I desperately did not want to become her.

How did you navigate intimacy with other partners after your rape?

I think that because I didn't want to end up like my mother, I did everything I could to do the opposite. For me at the time, that meant pretending that I was fine. I actually told myself and others that I liked being raped. I was so intent on it not affecting me that I really said that! It comes as no surprise that I surrounded myself with people who took advantage of me, and I was raped multiple time after the first assault, but I wouldn't admit it to myself because "I was fine." I was constantly trying to prove to myself that being abused didn't hurt. I was in a constant state of self-harm and repeating my trauma. This was such a low point for me. I was completely out of control. As I look back on this time of my life, this is where I have the most hurt and shame. The people that I chose to be around were the worst of the worst, and they did horrible and disgusting things to me and my body. At the time, I remember taking ownership of their actions; I was so desperate to convince myself that no one could hurt me that I told myself, "No, I am putting myself in these situations, so really they aren't hurting me . . . I am letting them do these things to me, so really I am the one in control." This went on for about six years.

You are now a mother with two small children. How did being pregnant and delivering a baby affect your feelings about your body?

Becoming a mother to two beautiful boys has been the biggest turning point for me in accepting my past and seeing my body in a more reverent light. I loved being pregnant, and I loved giving birth. The amount of forgiveness that I allowed myself to accept during that time was powerful. I never thought I would be blessed with babies because I didn't think that I deserved to be a mom, and I was, again, afraid of being a mom like my mother. I was shocked at how easily I slipped into the role of a mom. I think the universe in all its wisdom knew that motherhood was going to be my biggest tool for stepping into true self and seeing my body for what it really is. It is definitely something that I struggle with, especially since part of my self-harm involved cutting my skin, so I have scars all over my body. I am terrified of how I will have that conversation with my sons when they ask about what happened. I think it has shifted my focal point from the scars on my arms and legs and focused it on my heart and my boobs! My youngest is still breastfeeding, so a lot of my energy is absorbed in that. I consider it such a blessing to have reminders at all hours of the day and night that yes, your body is powerful. Yes, your body is strong. Yes, your body is needed in a pure and loving way.

What self-care worked for you in healing and feeling whole again?

I tried anything and everything, from traditional therapy to yoga and energy movement. All helped me along the way, but nothing I learned really sank in until I became a mom. I want to be an example of a strong, healthy woman to my boys so they grow up and know how to treat women. I want them to feel good in their skins, so I know I have to be their example. We dance, hug, and kiss, howl at the moon in our underwear; they play with painting their bodies and roll around in the dirt. If it brings a smile to their faces, then I want to give them the space to experience it. The best therapy has been having to show up every minute of every day to be the example that I wanted when I was a kid.

If you could speak to your younger self who experienced the assault, what would you tell her?

You are not your mother. Sometimes we need an example of what not to do to know what is right for our soul.

Anything else you would like to add?

Although I know I have a long way to go in fully healing my relationship with my body and being comfortable in sexuality, I think really embracing my relationship with shame completely dissolved the power it had over me. I now feel more in everything I do because I don't have this dark veil over me, causing me to doubt and criticize my need to be loved and to feel love.

Chapter 12

FOR MY SISTER

By Lyndsey Jones

Sister, you are the essence and embodiment of divine feminine.

Sister, you are grace, you are tenderness, you are power, you are strength.

Sister, set all that was once known aside, you are set free.

Sister, you embrace your new way of being. You are embracing your higher self, you are embracing your self.

Sister, you are speaking up and speaking out,

Sister, you are speaking your truth.

Sister, let me be your voice. Let me show you the passage to confidence, self-love, courage, and standing up.

Sister, we'll march together, hand in hand together. We can do this.

Sister, this story is for you.

Sister, this story is for me.

They sat there laughing so hard tears were running down their faces. Where she had gotten this sass, they weren't sure, but she was funny. Their laughing got me going more, waving my finger at them, telling Devon he needed to shape up, nagging at him like I was his parent. I don't remember ever seeing anyone do this to him, but I put on quite the comedy show.

My mom was a single parent with three kids to take care of, and she supported us with three jobs. My brother and I were with my aunt and uncle a lot. Their son, Devon, was like my older brother. I thought nothing of it when Devon asked Stephen and me who wanted to take a shower. I looked at Stephen, "Do you want to?"

He responded no, but I said, "I do I do!" I went into the bathroom. We got undressed; I remember feeling uneasy about this, uneasy about my body and being naked. I realized I hadn't ever showered or taken a bath with Devon, who was at least ten years older than me. He said, "Now you have to put this in your mouth before you can get in." He instructed me to not use my teeth and told me what to do. "You're doing it wrong," he said. I was embarrassed so I asked to get dressed. I didn't want to take a shower anymore. I was four.

I remember my mom yelling and my uncle holding her back. They made Devon apologize to me. "I don't know why you think this happened, but I'm sorry that you do," he said.

After that, my aunt couldn't take care of me anymore, even though we begged her to help. This started a path of bad babysitters and violations to my body, heart, mind, and soul. I lived most my life thinking I'd had a bad dream, lied, and torn my family apart.

I did stay there sometimes after Devon was out of the house. I started having nightmares of spiders coming out of the floor and a witch coming to get me. I started peeing on the floor instead of in the bathroom and got whipped for it. I have a vivid image of that witch coming through the door and standing in front of the toilet. It was the bathroom where that incident happened.

Sister, this is for the little sister who used to sing and dance to express joy, and now pain.

Sister, you played in silliness and giggles, and then fear and shyness.

Sister, this is for my sister who had her soul, her purity, her love, her passion, and her confidence taken too early.

Sister, this is for you who were told to wear your smile, to hide the darkness and shame.

It was late, dark outside, and dark inside. I was six.

The babysitter, Brenda, had served me hotdogs again, forcing me to eat every bite even though she knew I hated them. She had a scary movie on the television—I looked away. Refusing to finish my hotdogs, I was sent to the other room by myself. I stomped through the house and began screaming angry, sobbing cries. The next thing I remember is blood running down my face and shirt. Brenda had hit me so hard in the face that my nose was bleeding, and it had knocked me out for a second. Brenda and her 13-year-old daughter taunted and laughed at me standing over me in the bathroom, as I cried and cleaned my face in the mirror.

To this day, I hate hotdogs and Garth Brooks because of Brenda.

One night when my mom had a date, we stayed all day and night with Brenda. She would torture us by making us watch scary movies. She made me go to the grocery store to pick up a movie; they had decided on one called *Body Parts*. I prayed all the way there that it'd be out of stock. I think she ended up getting *Pet Sematary*, because *Body Parts* was nowhere to be found. When it was time for bed, I grabbed Stephen's hand for him to come to bed with me, but she ripped us apart. She made me sleep alone in her daughter Crystal's bed. She left the windows open above the bed. I cried and prayed that no one would kidnap me and slept with my eyes open until late.

Crystal would sometimes be left alone to watch us. She would make me take off my clothes or bring over dress-up clothes, and she would make Stephen and me watch her striptease, wearing my dress that didn't fit her and my underwear around her chest, exposing her nipples. She would come grab our faces when we turned away and make us watch her.

One 4th of July we were left with Brenda. Brenda and Crystal told us our mother didn't love us, or she'd be spending the 4th of July with us instead of her boyfriend. That was the first time we told our mother anything Brenda was doing or saying to us. She immediately removed us and took us to another babysitter, whose son would beat Stephen up. It wasn't any better.

The new babysitter couldn't take us in the evenings, so our Mom took us back to Brenda. The second time was worse than the first; that's when we started being threatened and told to stay quiet. We complained about the food to our mom and told her that other parents would bring groceries over to feed the kids Brenda watched after school.. So my single mom with three kids started bringing bags of groceries over, too. We never ate that food. We were forced to eat bland and insipid foods like hotdogs, beans and spaghetti and drink powdered milk. I stopped eating all together and started stashing my food under a place in the carpet.

One night Brenda served us spaghetti noodles covered in water and peppers, and she praised me for clearing my plate. I stared at my brother, begging him not to tell where my food was going. She sat next to him, telling him she was going to watch him eat every bite. He talked back and told her no. This made her angry and she lifted his plate, yelling, "If you're not going to eat it, you're going to wear it!" and crashed the glass plate over his head, shattering it.

When I was around age eight, my mom finally allowed my brother and me to stay home alone. We felt safer fending for ourselves than being left with people who were supposed to give us safety and protection.

Sister, this is for you, sister, who has been disregarded, ignored, pushed to the side.

Sister, did you think you were not allowed to talk about that pain or to remove the smile from that pretty face or show your tears?

Sister this is so you can find your beauty, peace, and love again.

Sister, I believe in you, even when you don't think you can believe in you.

Diana was our frizzy-haired, big glasses, bright-red-lipstick-wearing Sunday school teacher. She probably shouldn't have been teaching a young children's class. She shared stories about her shortcomings, divorce, and problems with alcoholism. "We all fall short, we're all sinners," Diana said. She would tell us that we were not good, and we never would be, and we needed to ask Jesus into our hearts. She spent the entire hour drilling this into us. When class was over I ran up to my mom and sobbed. I was so worried to tell her what a sinner I was that I didn't say anything, I just cried. I was nine.

I would ask Jesus into my heart every night. I'd lie in bed crying and begging to be rescued. I was sure the things that had happened to me were my fault, and they would eternally keep me separate from God. I lived in fear—scared of my body, scared of the secrets, scared of the shame in my heart.

Sister this story is for you my adolescent sister, starting to see your body differently, to having to cover it and protect it from hands that are not your own.

Sister did you have something stolen from you?

Sister let me offer it back to you.

Sister, you no longer have to be afraid, you can stand up straight, you can kick and cartwheel to honor your goodness and cheer.

Henry swept my mom off her feet; he swept us all off our feet. He had a big house in the country. It was like paradise. We were like a happy family playing games, playing fetch with our new dog and watching movies on a big TV screen—just never scary ones.

When we moved into the house, they were engaged to be married. Once we moved in, there were so many fights, and my mother often pulled me into them. She knew that Henry would stop verbally abusing her when I was around because he had a sweet spot for me.

Mom would work late at her retail job, and we were left with Henry. He used to play tag with us. We enjoyed the attention but then he started being kind of weird. He started being protective of me, while Stephen and I would play, and would get violent and physical with Stephen. He'd have me come down stairs and use his toothbrush, or run baths for me. Then he started having me cuddle in his bed. One night, he lifted my shirt and rubbed the skin under my shirt. I was ten.

When we moved into Kenny's house, we moved to a new school. Stephen and I were two out of a class of about fifteen students. It was the first time I actually felt popular, everyone was excited to have new students in the class, and at the school. The lunch lady made food from the local farmers, and we had some of the best lunches ever. I made friends with Carrie and I loved spending time at her house. Unless my mom was home, I didn't want to go home.

At some point, I went to visit my Aunt, the same one I used to stay with. I felt safe enough to tell her what was happening, and that I didn't feel safe with Henry. Suddenly, I was moving again. My mom moved us into a two-bedroom apartment, where I shared a room with my mom, and my brother had his own room.

Sister, this is for my teen sister who didn't get to choose when her flower was taken, she only awakened with a throb in her throat and her womb that couldn't be explained.

Sister I've heard that trauma is held in your cells for years after; betrayal of your body is soaked into your pores like a sponge.

Sister, let me show you there is light above your hopelessness.

Sister, find your sisterhood and nurture and have patience while you heal through your trauma.

When I was twelve, my mom got married to the man I call my Step-Dad, still today. We had a house of so much tension. It was a new experience for everyone, a house with two teenagers, and a new living situation for everyone. We were thrown into a house with a man, who would be a permanent part of our life, and that was not something we were used to. We were again in a different school. I was new, and was so frightened of life and god damnation that I couldn't open my mouth to even say hello.

I tried to hang on to my Christian roots when I left for college, very few friends or family in church supported me going to a non-Christian college, following my dream of art. I took a 4th year level class called Jesus. I decided that if this secular educational class could convince me my faith was worth holding onto, this would be it. Over the past year or so I had been brought to physical limits of not sleeping for days, I had several deaths in the family and friends, and had learned some things about family and friends that went against everything I thought I had learned from my Christian faith. I even got to a point where I took a bunch of sleeping aids to try and end my life. I decided that if this God I'd been giving all my love, time and energy to and begging to save my soul, if He didn't love me because of what adults had forced on me, I didn't want any of it.

It was about a year after I had made the lousy attempt to end my life; I was dealing with those same lousy feelings again. I was waking up have vivid nightmares and delusions of my sin turning into a sickness taking over my body. I was extremely depressed, and trying to figure out this body I had lost connection to years ago. I started painting this on the canvases in art class. I was spilling my secrets to strangers—they weren't ready, neither was I. I tried to get help at the school counselor's office. I sat for several hours waiting to be called. Finally, I walked out and kept on walking.

Sister, please allow yourself patience and time to recover from this. To come back to the altar that is inside all of you, where fear does not exist—a place of peace, love, happiness, purity, and joy.

"I am an adult survivor of childhood abuse, and I need help."

Saying this sounded so unreal, foreign, like I was betraying the mask I was told was required of me to be looked at as normal, as worthy, as valid. My body and my spirit were taken when I was four, then again when I was eight, and then again at ten, and then again at twelve, then again at twenty-one. It was a pattern I didn't ask for, yet I kept hearing I was the one doing something wrong. I haven't quite found my happy ending, but I have found power inside of me as I write down my truth.

My liberator is not found through religion, art, or any person. No longer staying quiet frees me.

Sister, you are love, you are loved, you are becoming the person you want to fall in love with.

Sister you are courageous, you are perfectly made, you are enough, you are worthy.

Sister, bound by fear, that freedom seems unreachable. Your voice cracks and you can't bear to make eye contact because god forbid someone see the pain you've survived and the power you have, standing strong, keeping your composure through it all.

Sister, this is for you who forgives and understands that it's okay to not forget.

Sister, forgiving isn't denying self or the trauma that has seeped into your cells.

Sister, you are ready to stop feeling like a fraud, an imposter, and acting like you're interested in the things you don't have an interest in. You are ready to be transparent and show the true color of your spirit and soul.

Sister, as you have aged you have found what brings light to your heart and what brings sadness to your heart.

Sister, with gray streaks in your hair, with your crown straight, with your head held high . . .

The cracks under your eyes show the joy in your smile, sister.

About the Author

Lyndsey Jones

What did you want to be when you were eight years old?

When I was eight, I wanted to be a princess and an artist.

If you could give one piece of advice to your younger self about your orgasm, what would it be?

You are beautiful and lovely and perfect in every way possible. It is your orgasm, it is your body, it is your power, and it is your choice! You are valid, and loved, you are enough and worthy.

If your orgasm had a voice, what would your orgasm say to you about the piece you wrote for this book?

YES, QUEEN!

Anything else you would like to add about your story or the experience of writing it?

This is the first time I am sharing my story, and am excited to share it in hopes I can bring light to someone else who needs to hear that they were born a queen.

ACKNOWLEDGEMENTS

Thank you to all the writers featured in this book for writing about events in their lives, especially the moments that felt too private to tell but that you wrote down anyway. Through your stories, we remember that our lives matter and that love is always present, even in the times when we felt the most alone, abandoned or betrayed. Your stories show us how you danced the path back to yourselves and remind us that we can find our way home, too.

Thank you to Paul Yinger for the beautiful cover designs for this book. Thank you for making my Os look so good.

Thank you to Dr. Liz Orchard for being a valued expert on women's bodies and wellness. Thank you for adding your words to the foreword of this book.

Thank you to the exceptional souls (both people and animals) at Chateau de Clerac in France where much of this book was edited during a writing retreat.

Thank you to my fantastic copy editor Amanda Coffin.

Made in the USA
Columbia, SC
22 August 2017